How To Experience More Joy And Less Stress Through Sustainable Farm Living
(Second Edition)

By Leigh and Olin Funderburk

With Paul Deepan

Foreword by Dan Miller

NY Times Best-Selling Author of

48 Days to the Work You Love

Original Copyright © 2016 Leigh and Olin Funderburk

Second Edition Copyright © 2018 Leigh and Olin Funderburk

Published by My Content Matters, LLC. All rights reserved.

ISBN-10: 1727467590
ISBN-13: 978-1727467598

DEDICATION

We would like to dedicate this book to our wonderful families, who gave us unconditional love, taught us the value of hard work, and forgave us our many transgressions throughout the years. We are blessed to have all of you in our lives and dearly miss those who have passed on. We would not have been able to write this book without all of you. Thank you for believing in us.

CONTENTS

Acknowledgments	i
Foreword By Dan Miller	Pg. 1
1. Introduction	Pg. 4
2. What Is Sustainable Farming, Anyway?	Pg. 15
3. Location, Launching, and Living	Pg. 21
4. Why Are You Doing This?	Pg. 36
5. Growing Healthy Food	Pg. 52
6. The Buzz About Bees	Pg. 81
7. Animals For Fun, Food and Profit	Pg. 92
8. Your Farm As Your Business	Pg. 132
9. Last Words	Pg. 158
About the Authors	Pg. 160

ACKNOWLEDGMENTS

As people of faith, we would like to acknowledge and thank God for the soft whispers to our hearts, which helped us discern and live out our farming and teaching vocation.

For his more earthly guidance, we would like to thank Dan Miller, author of *48 Days to the Work You Love*, for helping us discover our passion, and bringing it to life. We also acknowledge Dave Ramsey, author of *Financial Peace*, for sharing the principles that have helped us live a more sustainable, less "stuff-filled" life. The grass really does feel different under your feet when you are debt free!

Thanks also to Greg Latza for allowing us to use his photograph, which he shot at our farm, for the cover of this book. You can learn more about Greg's work by visiting www.greglatza.com

Finally, we thank Paul Deepan, author of, among other works, the wonderful novel *The Fruit of the Dendragon Tree*. Our collaborator and true friend, Paul's vision and experience across many writing genres and audiences helped breathe life into this book, and infuse it with our voices, so that we could authentically share our passion with you.

FOREWORD

A quick search for the term "rich" on Google brings up 859 million sites. Amazon shows 84,401 books with "rich" in the title. Obviously, it's a term that is on the mind of a whole lot of people. Thousands of songs have been sung about the benefits of being rich. In the classic movie *Fiddler on the Roof*, Tevye tells the world:

"If I were a rich man.
I wouldn't have to work hard…"

Madonna reminded us that:

"Only boys who save their pennies
Make my rainy day
'Cause we're living in a material world
And I am a material girl."

Little kids dream of growing up and being a sports, movie or music star so they can be rich and drive the car of their dreams. People tolerate jobs that don't fit their passions because "at least I'm making a living". And in the American dream that "living" will lead to a time of retirement where no productivity will be required. The earned reward will be time spent basking in the self-indulgent enjoyment of money that has been accumulated.

Yes, being "rich" is a very common theme.

And yet there's a new kind of "rich" that is creeping into the language of all generations. *I just want to be able to do what I love* is a bigger motivator for finding and choosing work than the assurance of a company car and 401K contribution. *I want to be able to make a difference in the world* is a more common mantra of a millennial than insistence on a corner office. Baby Boomers are discovering the power and fulfillment of relationships as being more valuable and lasting than stock portfolios that can disappear overnight. The fragility of what people thought was wealth has caused the younger generation to redefine what it means to be rich. Maybe it's not a bigger house or another vacation or a flashier diamond ring, but something more intangible and permanent – protected from the stock market variations and need for bank vaults and locked doors.

One dictionary definition of being rich describes it as having a large amount of something that is wanted or needed.

And that opens the door to the concept of being "Dirt Rich."

What if we understood being rich as sharing life with neighbors, being kind to the land we live on and showing good stewardship of the abundant resources we are privileged to enjoy? Could it be possible that a pot of soup made with fresh vegetables from the garden, enjoyed with friends from across the creek could be as valuable as a 5-star dinner in Paris? Is it possible that our kids would value time spent with us on a walk through the woods more than the guarantee of a paid for college education? Or that a porch swing made from an old discarded door would be even more beautiful than the latest model shipped across states from Henrodon in North Carolina? Is it imaginable that a simple painting done by a friend or grandchild would bring more joy to your home than the original Picasso (Nude, Green Leaves and Bust) that recently sold for $106.5 million?

In *Dirt Rich*, Leigh and Olin Funderburk lay out a beautiful plan for a simple, sustainable life style. Not one that strips the joy and beauty from life, but one that enhances those very characteristics. They guide us through their model of enriching their lives and those of the people in their community, and how you can do the same.

Olin and Leigh teach families where their food comes from, and introduce them to a place to relax, sit for a while in the rocker on the porch, visit the chickens and the goats and rediscover the natural beauty right in our back yards.

They share the thrill of growing and the enhanced nutrition of fresh vegetables, the challenges of growing fruit trees in harmony with animals, and the sheer joy of gathering wholesome brown eggs from healthy, free range chickens.

Dirt Rich serves as a reminder to each of us that our work is our ministry, acknowledging God's best gifts to each of us. Being rich is not the absence of work, but rather working with joy and purpose. We all have opportunities to be connected to each other, to the outdoors (what they call God's own cathedral) and to the abundance that living in this world provides. We are responsible for seeing our land not as something belonging to us but as a community we can nurture, share and pass on to future generations.

And yes, in doing so, we can all be Dirt Rich.

~ Dan Miller

1. INTRODUCTION

If you are reading these words, it's possible you are yearning, as we were, for a life less filled with stress and anxiety, and one that is more filled with meaning. You might be willing to give up a bite out of your income for a taste of freedom. You might be willing to trade status for simplicity. You might be ready to take the plunge and buy a piece of rural property and become farmers. Even if not, you might consider homesteading on your own property, as far as the local laws might permit, and even if all you are able to do is build a square foot garden, or a vertical one hanging from a railing or fence, we hope that some of the insights we share with you in this book will be helpful.

When we first thought it might be a good idea to write a book, we didn't really know how to go about doing it. Both of us can write, but that didn't mean we could write a book, especially about our own journeys. But we weren't deterred, because when we started our farm, we didn't know all that much about sustainable farming, either. Both of us grew up on and around farms, but sustainable farming, especially on one as small as ours, is different from traditional farming. The business focus of our farm is also very different to the farms we worked on during our early lives.

But we've learned in our journey together that sometimes you just have to take that calculated risk, and to listen to that inner voice that tells you to do something a little outside of your comfort zone, and that if you do it with the right intention, the help you need along the way will be provided. Starting a farm can feel overwhelming, so hopefully, for you, this book will be a little piece of that help. Just as it did when we started our farm, the help for writing this book did appear, and here we are. We wanted to share some of the things we've learned about sustainable farm living, so that maybe your road to that life we've come to love becomes a little more accessible, a little more realistic, and has a few more signposts.

When we started our farm, we didn't really know what our real passion and purpose was, and only discovered these through trial and error a few years into the process. This might seem a little backwards, especially given our skeptical, even cynical society. But we can definitely tell you today that our passion is to teach people how to achieve the deep satisfaction that that comes from learning how to grow healthier food, and from using the land in a sustainable way. We have become teachers of a way of life that affords the feel of dirt under your nails, and earth under your feet. We teach the contentment of living a life that feeds you and your loved ones, as well as how to make a living, while living with that contentment.

We certainly didn't know, when we started, that the mission of our farm was going to be about teaching others how to farm, and how to help others rediscover healthy, needful skills and practices that are becoming increasingly rare in our materialistic, consumer society. As people of faith, we believe that God has had much to do with bringing us to this destination, not just of place, but of purpose. But people from all over the world come to our farm for the nurturing it provides, and you don't have to believe as we do to share the same desires for simplicity and meaning that we have.

And you don't have to know all the answers to all the questions before you begin your journey: a lot of success, certainly a lot of our success, has to do with having the courage to take that first step along the path.

So let's walk together for a time, shall we?

Never Say Never Again (Leigh's Story):

A lot of people who visit Stoney Creek Farm ask me what I did to prepare myself for a life of sustainable farm living. Some of my friends and visitors only know that I had a career in corporate America, most recently with Xerox, and of course it would be easy to be confused about how a sales career with Xerox might prepare one for a life on the farm!

Some people would say that I had a tough childhood, but I believe that God uses all circumstances for His good and His purpose. My childhood helped to make me stronger and shape me into the person that I am today. I was born in Humboldt Tennessee, but moved to Texas when I was 2 years old. My mother and father unfortunately had marital difficulties, which ultimately ended in their separation and divorce, and my mother eventually moved my brother and me back to Tennessee so that she could raise us around her supportive family. Mom was the oldest of 11 children, with her youngest sister only 3 years older than me. My grandparents, aunts, and uncles were very good to us and provided wonderful role models for my brother and I to look up to.

During this time, we lived on a small farm rented to us by my mother's sister and brother-in-law. My brother and I learned how to work on the farm in the large garden that we had behind the house. That garden provided a substantial amount of food for our family that we could not have done without. My mom's job only paid minimum wage, so that garden made a huge difference in how well we ate throughout the year. We also learned farm work from Uncle Brance and Aunt Joyce, who let us work for them by chopping weeds out of the cotton fields. It was hot, hard work that taught me the value of a dollar and kept me out of trouble. It also motivated me to go to college so that I did not have to do farm work the rest of my life. I specifically remember telling my family "I will never, ever marry a farmer or live on a farm."

You never should say: "Never;" God has a way of making you eat your words.

As a typical teenager, I would have said I hated working in the garden, chopping weeds, or canning vegetables, but there are some things I remember now that bring back a lot of great memories… my mama's candy pickles, canned green beans, purple hull peas, grape jelly, and peaches. If we hadn't moved back to Tennessee I would've never learned all the wonderful things that my mother taught me, in the summers during the garden season. I still remember all the smells of pickling, blanching, and canning all the wonderful fruits of our labor.

In Tennessee, I was able to make the deep-rooted relationships I'd missed during our nomadic days in Texas. Mom took us to church every Sunday, and I know that my faith has brought me through some difficult times.

My mother insisted that we go to college. She did not want us working minimum wage jobs, like she was forced to do after she and my father split up. Since we didn't have a lot of money, I knew that I needed to get scholarships to be able to go to college. So I worked hard and because of my grades I received several scholarships that allowed me to attend Middle Tennessee State University in Murfreesboro Tennessee, although I still had to work (more than one job) during college. After I graduated, I had several job offers, and I took the one that paid the most, as a Kroger store manager trainee starting at $19,000 per year, which was not bad money at all for a young woman fresh out of college in the 80s. Kroger at that time was promoting women and diversity in their stores and corporate office so I had an eight-year career with them, first in store management and later in floral merchandising.

In Kroger's excellent management training program, I learned how to cut meat, merchandise the store, and ensure food safety, human resource skills, inventory control, and relationship management with the union. Retail hours were not fun but I advanced quickly and thoroughly enjoyed my career. One of the most memorable experiences I had was being able to visit all of the floral growing areas in California. I flew into San Francisco and the Wesco rep drove us down the coast all the way to San Diego. I not only learned a lot about the floral business but I also learned a lot about produce being grown in California. I had never seen artichokes or avocados growing in the field until that trip.

During my tenure at Kroger, I lost my mother to a sudden, fatal heart attack. She was only 47 years old. I cannot tell you how much that event has shaped my life from that point on. I was very close to my mother, who had devoted her whole life to raising my brother and me in the best way she knew how. I was 24 when she died and the void that was left in my heart could never be filled. Time and faith has healed my wounds, but there is not a day that goes by that I don't think of her and her many sacrifices to make sure our family stayed together. I learned that every day is a gift from God and I want to honor her and our family by living life to the fullest and serving others...a meaningful legacy that she would be proud of.

Shortly after my mother passed away, I married and five years later had my daughter. I realized that retail hours were not conducive to family life. Sometimes I would close the store at midnight and have to be back the next morning at 6 AM so it didn't take long to get sleep deprived, especially with a newborn. So I started looking at some of the vendors for Kroger for possible job opportunities and found the plant manager position at a regional fresh vegetable processing facility. This position afforded me regular hours and a more flexible schedule with my newborn daughter. The food processing plant helped me to learn about production requirements, quality control, tight inventory turn and much more. After three years in plant management, I moved into a regional marketing director position, and learned valuable marketing skills such as branding, sales, and customer relationship management. I also had the privilege of rolling out a new product line, which was fresh fruit that would last 10 days with no preservatives. The process was unique and involved boiling the fruit (like cantaloupe and honeydew) for a specified amount of time to kill all bacteria on the fruit's outer skin. The boiling time was critical so that it did not cook the fruit. It was a total secret because we could not patent the process and we didn't want competitors finding this out.

During my marketing director term, I discovered that the owners of this regional company were positioning it for sale nationally, so I began searching for another career, and was eventually hired into a corporate sales position with Xerox. Xerox definitely had one of the best sales training programs in the country, and I was blessed to have the opportunity to work there. This was hard work of a different kind, but I stuck it out and developed a successful career path over the next 17 years. I started out as an account manager working with a local territory and ended up as a production sales specialist covering parts of seven states. The large ticket equipment I sold yielded a very generous compensation package...for which I felt very blessed.

During my 17 years at Xerox, I went through a divorce, continued to raise my daughter (with a lot of help from her father), then met and married my soul mate, Olin Funderburk, and, despite my earlier promise to never find myself back on a farm, moved with him, all but 'kicking and screaming', to a small 15 acre farm in Williamson County, Tennessee.

The Frog Prince (Olin's Story):

I was born in Biloxi Mississippi at the Keesler Air Force base, where my Dad was stationed at the time. We moved to Seminary, MS when my mother got a teaching job there. And by the way, yes, Seminary is the real name of that very little town, which is in Covington County, MS, and was named after the Zion Seminary, which was formed in 1845.

Because both of my parents worked, my grandparents helped care for me on their farm until I was about two years old. My grandparents raised dairy and beef cattle and grew soybeans, corn, and other row crops. We moved to Santa Susanna, California, when I was two, because my Dad was promised a job by my uncle who lived there. Not long after, though, we moved again because my Dad, Carl, felt called to plant new churches in California, and I guess in a way he was a farmer of sorts too, except his harvest was souls.

We ended up In Barstow, CA, which has a marine base nearby where Dad worked. My Mom taught Home Economics at Barstow High School, while Dad started a church plant. In the summers, I'd spend time back in Mississippi on my grandparent's farm, and those of my aunts and uncles. I really enjoyed those summers working on the farm and being close to family.

In 1968, we moved to New Orleans, so that my Dad could attend seminary (for one year), and then he was called to a church in Brookhaven, Mississippi, which is about 55 miles west of Seminary. I still spent my summers back at the farm with my grandparents, helping them with the dairy and the row crops. I was very close to my grandparents, and I guess because I loved the farm so much I became something of a favorite grandchild with them, which caused a certain amount of ribbing from my cousins.

In 1975, my Dad received a call to serve as a pastor in Springfield, South Carolina. Those summers, I worked with local farmers during the summers until I graduated high school in 1977. It shouldn't be surprising by this time that I decided I wanted to go to college in MS, and live with my grandparents. So I started at Jones Junior College in 1977, where I completed my Associate's degree. My grandfather died from lung cancer in May 1979, and I stayed on with my grandmother through the fall of 1981 to help her with the farm, and to go to school.

My grandmother's oldest daughter, Olene, came to live with her that fall, so I moved into an apartment with my best friend, Jeff Ford. By this time, I was attending the University of Southern Mississippi in Hattiesburg, attending college full time, while also working full time in an auto body shop to pay my way through school. I graduated college in 1982 with a BS in Construction and Engineering. I worked for two construction companies in Mississippi during this time, and in the same period I got married. All the while, I kept searching for other career opportunities, and ended up in Tennessee working for the THDA Housing Authority from 1987-1996. Our family grew bigger with a great source of joy…our two sons, Lin and Landry.

In 1996, a private construction company approached me to help them develop additional THDA opportunities, and I joined them for the next ten years. In 2006, four of us who worked for this company, formed a partnership and bought the company we worked for. Today there are three separate entities under this partnership: engineering, property management, and construction.

Life isn't always smooth sailing though, and between 1998 and 2000 my wife and I separated and eventually divorced. I met my current wife Leigh in 2001, through two mutual friends, Judy and Linda, who thought we would make a good couple. I'd already dated a few women since my divorce, so was already interested in meeting Leigh, but she hadn't had such a positive experience since her own divorce, and that negative reinforcement from dating a few "frogs" made her reluctant to meet me.

Leigh thought of as "frogs" men who, no matter how much you kiss them, don't turn into princes. And like I said because Leigh had met a few of these it took a while for our two matchmakers to get Leigh to go out with me. One day in January 2001, Judy came to Leigh's house with a newspaper picture to show her what I supposedly looked like. The picture was of Jeff Fisher, who at the time was the head coach of Nashville's NFL team, the Titans. Leigh thought Jeff Fisher was a pretty handsome guy (and I can't argue), so she agreed to go to lunch with me in Nashville.

I called her the week before our date and to her surprise (Leigh later told me) we talked for 45 minutes on the phone. It became clear we had a lot in common, both our childhoods being spent on farms, strong among them. Two years later, we walked down the aisle together, soul mates then, and soul mates now.

When we decided to buy the property that is now Stoney Creek Farm, where we live, Leigh wasn't exactly enthusiastic. Although she'd been raised on a farm, or, maybe, because she'd been raised on a farm, she'd told her family when she left to go to college that she wouldn't ever marry a farmer, or live on a farm, ever again. Well, she'd already married me, so I thought the next step wouldn't be so hard, but I had to get very creative to persuade her to take the leap back to the farm with me.

I guess even though it was, and is, hard work, I'd never lost my love of farming that I first had from those early years working on my grandparent's and relative's farms. The respect I have for the land, and the deep satisfaction that only comes from a job well done through hard work, stayed with me all my life. I could always see these same qualities in Leigh, and I always believed that once I got her "back to the dirt" that she would recognize where these traits really came from, and fall in love with the land again the way I'd always been in love with it.

I'd say maybe she has.

How I Fell in Love with our Farm (Leigh again):

So yes, OK, Olin's right, and I have to admit that despite coming here all but kicking and screaming, I did fall in love with the place immediately. A creek with a stone bed winds almost through the entire farm, and lends its identity to the name of our property: Stoney Creek Farm. In the spring we have about a quarter acre of yellow daffodils (otherwise known as buttercups) growing all around the creek. In the summer the native Yucca plants bloom a field of white. We are abundantly rich with native wildlife, trees and plants and it's a beautiful and peaceful place to live.

Our residence is actually a pole barn design, complete with steel beams and stained concrete floor, finished inside as a house. Olin has always enjoyed repurposing and recycling materials, and this barn/house was the perfect experiment for him. One of our biggest conversation pieces is the pair of 100-year-old barn doors lining the dining room wall. He also built two full 12'x60' porches on the front and back of the barn for more outdoor living space, and a three car garage on the end of the barn with lots of room for a freezer, extra refrigerator and storage. Later, Olin finished the upstairs hayloft into a large bonus room, bedroom and third full bathroom in the barn.

This hybrid barn/house has proven to be comfortable, simple, and very sustainable. By building a pole barn with metal there is very little maintenance for at least 30 years. The only maintenance is replacement of the screws that hold the metal roof every 10 years.

The concrete floors are also very easy to maintain and keep clean. Olin also built a smaller barn and workshop with two more garage bays and horse stalls in the back. We determined that it was too much work and too much money for us to maintain our own horses, but sometime in the future we may be able to board horses as another source of income, so I'm glad we have the stalls.

We've experimented unsuccessfully with small fruit orchards (cedar rust and thieving raccoons) and meat goats (coyotes), but we still have a few goats for kids to pet when they come to visit, and may decide to breed again one day.

After these learning experiences, in 2011 we decided to offer rental gardens and a U-Pick Garden. In Williamson County there is a huge amount of people living in apartments, condos, and homes with small lots. We felt that many of these people would like to grow their own healthy food, and with our backgrounds in farming we were hoping that we could help them do so.

Our goal does not revolve solely around making money, it's about helping people to see the benefits of sustainable farm living - benefits which I call less stress, more joy. As a former participant in the rat race, I know the value of healthy living with lower stress, because my blood pressure went down almost immediately when I left Xerox to concentrate full-time on growing our sustainable farm model.

The farm has been full of surprises, allowing me to stretch my interests and create opportunities to teach those things no longer taught in schools, or even passed down in family traditions, things like Canning, Making Sourdough Bread, and much more. I have also taken painting classes and now sell paintings and teach painting (occasionally) at the farm. All these things simply bring us a great deal of joy, and we want to share our joy with you, whether you want to learn how you also can permanently get out of the corporate rat race, or just need a break from it on the weekend.

When people stop by and see us, they see their kids laugh as they play with our silly goats, miles away from the nearest video game. They tell us they can actually feel their bodies relaxing, as they walk among the flowers, picking vegetables outside in the fresh air, and not under fluorescent lights while freezing to death in the air-conditioned maze of some anonymous big box store. Many share how wonderful it feels to take their shoes off, and dig their feet into the "dirt wealth" that nourishes so many people, on so many levels. Whatever the reason for the city scowl they might have arrived with, they have a country smile by the time they leave.

2. WHAT IS SUSTAINABLE FARMING, ANYWAY?

The Philosophy of Sustainability

One of the questions we get a lot is: "What's Sustainable Farming? Is it like organic farming?" It's interesting to us that "Organic" Farming seems to have become synonymous with "Best Practice" Farming, and the way the question is posed typically reveals this bias that "organic" is the higher benchmark, and "sustainable," while nice, is a somehow inferior label. We don't mind this, as the organic industry has done a very good job of marketing itself as a superior option to the "regular" food you buy at the supermarket. And we think our food is superior as well. But we'd like to take a little time here to explain the differences, as becoming a "sustainable" farmer, which is what this book is trying to help you do, is a different thing entirely than becoming an "organic" farmer, and those differences are important to understand.

While there are some similarities between the two, when it comes to farming, sustainable and organic are not the same. We also think the sustainable label not only takes more discipline at the farming operation level, it will also have a more extensive impact on how you live your life in other ways. The National Organic Program (NOP) has developed several strict criteria regarding what constitutes an organic farm, but interestingly there are no such rules to ensure that organic farmers or organic food production operations follow ecologically sound practices, which is a large part of sustainability.

A lot of people prefer to buy food that is labeled "organic" but we think it's important to understand some of the limits of organic certification. As consumers and prospective farmers, you should probably know something about these limits, as well as the differences between organic foods and sustainable foods. As farmers and teachers of farm practices, we definitely need to know these differences, so that we can market our products honestly, and successfully educate our students as well.

1. "Sustainable" is not an official certification, but a mindset

Unlike "USDA Certified Organic" "Sustainable" is not a government-benchmarked label or official policy. Most people would probably describe sustainability as philosophy, one that encourages farming practices that help protect our planet, and which can be continued indefinitely without damaging the environment.

But just because we can't label the food we produce as "Sustainable," doesn't mean that "Sustainability" is just an abstract idea. Sustainable farm practices measurably improve a farm's and a community's economic profit, social benefits, and environmental protection.

2. Sustainable is Small, Diverse, and Non-Toxic

A sustainable farmer will tend to own less land and grow more diverse crops, which helps boost crop productivity and protection, enhances the soil and conserves land resources. A sustainable farmer might also try vertical planting, or other techniques designed for less space, and allow animals to graze on cultivated land.

One of the main criteria for organic farming involves the type of seed required. Certified organic farms can only use heirloom seed, which is not genetically diverse. This can result in plants that may not weather tough growing conditions, and which could be susceptible to common diseases. We use a combination of heirloom and hybrid seed (seed that is produced by cross-pollinated plants) at our farm, which helps with disease resistance and boosts production.

We also do not use GMO (Genetically Modified) seed, and stay away from pesticides, just like organic farms. We grow flowers to attract beneficial insects and use integrated pest management strategies... just like organic farms. We'll talk more about these practices in a later chapter.

While organic farmers may adopt some of these practices, a huge pumpkin farm, as an example could meet the definition of "Organic," but likely wouldn't be considered "sustainable." This is because a single-crop, large-acreage organic farmer could possibly use more land than necessary, waste resources such as water, and use (organic-approved) fertilizers, which bleed into the water table. Since land acreage, biodiversity, water consumption and fertilizer use are not covered by NOP policy, you can see how a large organic farmer may not be a sustainable farmer.

3. Sustainable is Water Efficient

As mentioned in the previous section, under NOPD policy, organic farmers or processors are not required to conserve water resources. On the other hand, sustainable farmers and processors do proactively try to conserve water.

Sustainable farming methods may include using reclaimed water (such as rain water, which we use almost exclusively) for some crops, planting drought-tolerant crop species, or using reduced-volume irrigation systems.

4. Sustainable is Energy Efficient

Most organic farms and food processing plants depend heavily on non-renewable energy sources, such as petroleum. While petroleum use is sometimes unavoidable, sustainable food farmers and processors understand that the continued use of non-renewable energy is, literally, unsustainable, so they will attempt when economically feasible to use alternative power sources such as wind, solar or water. We have done our own due diligence on alternative energy sources for Stoney Creek Farm, and although the economics currently don't allow us to use them, we are always evaluating ways to use more sustainable energy sources.

Locally grown organic food, which relied for its growth and distribution on alternative fuels such as ethanol or biodiesel, could be optimal from the standpoint of energy sustainability. But from the perspective of fossil fuel use only, "organics" can't generally compete with locally grown sustainable food.

This is because organic certification does not measure the "carbon footprint" of any fossil fuels used for food production or transport. Many organic food growers and companies ship their organic food products large distances from farm to warehouse, in vehicles that use traditional fossil fuels. The energy costs of both storing and distributing organic foods can therefore be significant.

5. Sustainable is More Humane to Animals

Many people today have concerns about the treatment of animals, especially in large farming operations. The humane treatment of animals is something any farmer can decide upon, but organic certification does not mean animals were treated decently. While the USDA's organic certification does include limited rules about animal access to pasture, but the USDA does not officially mandate animal welfare through NOP. This means that "organic livestock" can, for instance, spend much of their lives in confinement, with little thought given to their overall well-being.

In a sustainable livestock system, the farmer considers the wellbeing of livestock, and will typically provide as much outdoor space as necessary so that animals can root, peck or graze in a natural manner. When it's necessary to house animals indoors, a sustainable farm provides a more comfortable indoor space as well.

For instance, we have had to house our chickens in a coop overnight, due to predators, but this coop was built to allow the hens plenty of room to move about, and is appropriately cooled and heated in the summer and winter respectively. They also have an outdoor enclosure where they can roam about freely, and this is fenced off and covered with chicken wire to prevent depredation from hawks and other predators.

Coyotes preyed upon the kids from our initial goat family, and while we still have three adult goats, we continue to think how we can re-introduce young kids into a more protected environment. We are considering fostering a donkey for this purpose, as they are proven deterrents against coyotes. The feed cost for a foster animal is tax deductible, which makes sense for a small farm with a limited herd.

6. Sustainable means eco-friendly packaging

Sustainable food is food that is not only healthy for the people eating it, but also for the planet. This extends to decisions around food packaging. For example, you could grow organic strawberries, but then place them in tiny plastic bins, cover them with plastic shrink-wrap, and then pack everything in a bigger box. Such over-packaging is not eco-friendly.

Wherever possible, we try to use glass instead of plastic. Glass containers are fully recyclable, whereas plastic containers, although they may be partially recycled or repurposed, are made with non-renewable petroleum, and are less eco-friendly than glass ones. I mean, do you really recycle your shrink-wrap?

A sustainable packaging process uses the least amount of resources, with the highest available potential for recycling. Sustainable packaging should ideally be 100% recyclable and printed with eco-friendly inks as well. Not all certified organic food is packaged in such a sustainable manner.

7. Sustainable is not just about the food

Don't get us wrong: we are definitely not trying to knock organic farming, or farmers. An organic certification reflects a rigorous and disciplined commitment to meet government-regulated standards. It's just that you can totally meet "organic" standards and not necessarily operate your farm in a sustainable or even ethical way, because NOP rules don't cover such considerations.

Living on a smaller property with less "stuff "tends to lead to more sustainable living overall than a "more is better" lifestyle, since sustainability results from a need- based approach to consumption rather than a desire-based one.

Farming decisions based on sustainability will probably start to extend to other sustainable practices, such as a paperless (or reduced paper) office, using less gas-based transportation, protecting the immediate community beyond the farm borders, fair working conditions for employees and interns, and so on.

This is because adopting true sustainable farm practices will, all by itself, encourage you to think beyond your food or animal farming operations, into your management and individual goals and lifestyle choices. USDA organic policy doesn't cover much with regard to sustainable practices even at the farm operation level, so it's sure not going to encourage you to be more environmentally friendly in ways beyond how food is grown.

So when people ask us if Stoney Creek is an organic farm, or if our food is organic, we are actually proud to say we are not. Instead, we try to follow, as much as possible, a fully sustainable lifestyle, not only on our farm, but also in our daily lives.

3. LOCATING, LAUNCHING, AND LIVING

Location, Location, Location:

Let's assume you're ready to become a farmer. You've made the internal decision, probably over many months, that life in the country, while hard work, will give you a lot more inner satisfaction that what you may already be doing. You want to feel more joy, you want to have less stress, and you want to create more meaning, not only in your life, but also in the lives of your loved ones, and even the community around you.

Well, that's wonderful! We've made that transition, and we welcome you with open arms. So the first thing you may be wondering is, well, where am I going to have this farm?

The short answer to this question is: Location, location and location! That's right, this mantra is not just for city folks any more, and possibly was always more true for farmers than for, say, your favorite restaurants.

This chapter is to help you recognize some of the things you will need to think about when deciding where you are going to have your farm. If you have a life partner, it should hopefully go without saying that they support you in this dream. If they don't we would STRONGLY recommend getting that support before driving out to the country every weekend looking at potential farm properties.

As an aside, Olin still has a full time job in his own construction company, while Leigh is on the farm running the operation full time, with Olin's help as needed. Olin's particular situation means that he travels all over the place anyway, but if your partner has to go to a specific work destination most of the time, then their daily commute becomes an important part of the farm location decision.

Road Access:

As it happens, Stoney Creek is very close to local main roads and thoroughfares, which not only makes it easy for us to get to work-related meetings away from the farm, but also for the general public to find and visit us.

And yes, another thing you will want to ask yourself is whether you will want your farm to be open to the public. If so, and depending upon whether this access will be year round or seasonal, it will likely need to be fairly close to main roads so that the public can find and access your location.

However, this may not always be the case. For example, the Lucky Ladd Farm in Murfreesboro, Tennessee, is a seasonal "Destination Farm" that closes for the winter. Among other attributes, it has a Petting Zoo, as well as a lot of acreage, with nature trails and animals, and advertises over 70 activities for the entire family. Lucky Ladd is not close to main roads, but is a destination kind of place, and the "draw" of what they offer makes the drive worthwhile for the folks who visit them.

To run a "Destination" farm off the beaten path, you do need a big draw. For a U-Pick Garden such as ours, you'd need more than the two acres that we offer if you weren't close to a large urban center. If you wanted the public to come and view dairy goats, for example, you'd also need to be close. However if you just want to sell your goat cheese, etc. then you'd only need to be within travelling distance to market. (Be careful of the economics of this, as well. You should always factor in your fuel cost and vehicle mileage when calculating net profit on market sales).

Ideally, your farm should have frontage on the main road the public uses to visit you. Stoney Creek does not have such frontage, which in a perfect world we would prefer. Instead, we have an easement, and are fortunate to have good neighbors. We have friends who have easements on their less co-operative neighbor's land, and are not as easily able to have access. So you should also know who your neighbors will be, and check them out before you buy the land.

Land Cost:

In Middle Tennessee, land prices can vary widely even between two counties that are adjacent to each other. In Williamson County, which is just south of Nashville, and where we live, the excellent school system and relatively easy commute into downtown Nashville, has driven property prices very high, compared to, for example, next door Maury County. If property acquisition cost, and its impact on your budget, is something you want to manage (and it should be) you would want to also factor that in to your farm location decision.

Also, if the area you desire is on the more expensive side, you can determine exactly how much land you will need for your farm business and settle on a property with less acreage. Although there are tax advantages to having a farm above a certain size (which we will discuss later) we could probably operate our entire business model on less than 5 acres of land... you may need even less.

All this being said, if you find a property with which you fall in love, and it doesn't have a lot of access, you can still market your way to visibility, as visibility from the road is not always necessary for your business model. But if you have no road frontage and have an easement instead, you will need good neighbors.

Zoning:

One of the other major issues you need to consider when deciding upon your farm's location is the county zoning laws. Zoning is very important, because it may well dictate what you can and can't do!

Zoning laws can change without notice as well, so you may suddenly (without warning) find yourself at odds with the local zoning regulations, so it's important that you stay in compliance with them.

We advise that you go to your county planning commission (or go online) to find out what development, if any may be planned for the area where your prospective land is (plus current zoning, etc.). Also find out what the planned population for the county will be.

It's usually easy to get a copy of the local zoning ordinances for the area you are considering for purchase, since they are free to the public. We are able to pull up our county zoning ordinances online, which makes gathering the details very easy. Some zoning regulations prohibit "Agritourism," so it is extremely important that you know exactly what is allowed for your property...because re-zoning is a LOT more work than buying property that already has appropriate regulations for your business.

Launching:

There are significant tax advantages to being classified as a "Green Belt" farm, and, if you can afford the land cost, we would definitely encourage you to pursue this classification. The minimum size of a Green Belt farm varies by state, and 15 acres is the minimum in Tennessee. One requirement of this classification is to produce and sell $1,500 a year in "agricultural goods." This liberal classification can include lumber, hay, produce, cattle, chickens, and much more. Being a green belt farm can save a significant amount in property taxes. You can read more about "Green Belt" classification in the Tennessee Farm Bureau document found at this URL: http://www.tnfarmbureau.org/sites/default/files/greenbeltbrochure.pdf

This document describes the Green Belt classification as follows:

"The Greenbelt Law, or the Agricultural, Forest, and Open Space

Land Act of 1976, was designed to maintain farms, forests, and open space and reduce urbanization across Tennessee. Greenbelt helps provide tax relief, not exemption, to those who qualify." (TCA 67-5-1002)

According to Wikipedia, "A green belt or greenbelt is a policy and land use designation used in land use planning to retain areas of largely undeveloped, wild, or agricultural land surrounding or neighboring urban areas."

In addition to seeking greenbelt status (if possible), we feel it is important to earn an adequate income on your farm, if you plan on deducting expenses (such as depreciation) as a working farm. The IRS doesn't recognize "hobby farms" as real business models. That's why Leigh joined a local networking group: she needed to double the farm income and referrals from this group allowed her to do so. We'll talk more about the potential benefits of joining business networking groups when we discuss marketing in a later chapter.

You can depreciate used equipment as well. And you can buy lots of good used farm equipment on websites such as Craigslist. Be as appropriately aggressive as you can to get the main tax benefits of being a working farm. But, absolutely don't break the law, and don't take any deductions that could throw up a red flag, and get you audited.

Sustainable Housing:

Part of the reason we made the move to the country is because Olin doesn't do well with Home Owners Associations (we know, join the club, right?). Although Leigh had vowed never to move back to a farm, she agreed that if Olin could find a property to build a house on, and not increase our mortgage payment (with a 15 year term), then we would move. Leigh thought it was a pretty safe bet that Olin couldn't do this, but in 2005, the real estate market was very "hot" and contributed to his success.

Our realtor friend, Lisa Coe, had been approached about selling a neighbor's property, and in turn approached Olin about it. He was able to view it before it was listed on MLS and immediately offered to buy it. He was able to buy the land for about $50 more per month than the suburban home we had at the time, with a 15-year mortgage too! Today, in Williamson County, if you list your house in the morning it can be gone by the afternoon (good luck finding another one to move into though, but that's a different story.) Timing is everything.

Next, Lisa listed our home for more money than we thought it would bring, even in the 'hot' market, and sold it for list price in three days. The equity in our suburban home (plus a little extra) was enough to build our current home on the farm, so that we did not need an additional mortgage.

As we mentioned in the introduction, our house is really a pole barn design, which we have converted into usable living space with three bedrooms. When designing a house for a rural property, you must consider the position of the "Perc" site(s) on the land. Perc (or percolation) is the rate at which water absorbs into the ground, and is important to know for the septic system. The perc site and its size determine how many people can occupy the proposed home and the number of bedrooms. (In most states, a bedroom is considered a room with a closet). Two bedrooms will usually mean that you have a maximum of 4 people using the property, while a 3 bedroom, will imply a maximum of 6. The bathroom number is irrelevant, but you have to make sure (especially if you are building your house) about whether the septic site is downhill, or if you will have to pump it uphill. A septic system that has to use a pump will incur more cost.

When buying a property, you need to be aware, if you aren't already, that bank regulations around financing changed significantly after the financial crisis of 2008/09. It simply isn't as easy at it once was to obtain financing for a loan, even for an asset like real property.

You should know, if you are building, that your land will have to be no more than a third of the total property value. This is a general rule of thumb for conventional loans, but not a law or regulation. In other words, your house's value has to be twice the land's value. As an example, if you buy a $250K piece of land, you will have to have a house worth $500K. This is why houses are tending to get so big around where we are, because since land values in Williamson County have become so high, the square footage of the home now has to be large enough to satisfy the mandated valuation ratios of the land compared to the house structure.

To obtain financing for our purchase, we went to Farm Credit Services (https://www.fcsamerica.com), which is the oversight body for multiple farm credit organizations across the country. The liquidity for farm property loans comes from commercial investors who purchase debt securities (bonds) issued by the Federal Farm Credit Banks Funding Corp.

Farm Credit does not have the same general rules around their loans (e.g. house value twice the land value) that conventional mortgage companies do. The website for the association that serves Tennessee (and is part of the Farm Credit System), is https://e-farmcredit.com/home.

Farm Credit Mid America is the one we used, and is located in Dickson, TN. They were a truly great resource for us, and we would highly recommend them.

So, we bought the "dirt" and then we used the equity built up in our other house to place pay cash for the home on our farm.

We originally thought we would use the barn for a Bed & Breakfast or as a home for Olin's Mom and Dad later in their lives, so they could be near family, and we intended to build another home across the creek for us to live in. But in 2008, when the economy essentially fell off the cliff, and Olin's business (construction contractor) tanked, we re-thought our plan, and decided to stand pat with the building investment we already had.

We never wanted to be a "normal" Williamson Co. farm. One day Olin met with a guy he knew whose business was building pole barns. He wanted Olin to see a structure he was building for a lawyer in Brentwood. The lawyer's wife wanted something with a barn, stables, and living quarters, and we really liked the way the concept had panned out, so we started doing the numbers.

When you build a structure, wood is admittedly very pretty, but it needs a LOT of maintenance. Vinyl siding claims to be "maintenance free" but may only last about ten years before it starts cracking, etc. So we decided to build a metal barn with a metal roof as our house structure, and it truly is maintenance-free. The house is simply a standard "pole barn," in that poles hold up the building. These poles are set in the ground, then concrete is poured, and the structure built around it.

A metal structure can save you a lot on insurance as well, as it is generally a non-combustible material, termite-resistant, etc. We have full replacement value on our insurance, which is not always possible with other materials. It is important to check with your insurance agent about their policies concerning non-traditional structures, since these can vary a great deal.

Our house is set at 12 feet "on center," on a grid pattern. You can go bigger to have more open space, if you want. Our walls are six inches thick because we used 6 x 6 posts. Our insulation is good due to this thickness, and beats EPA recommendations.

You have many options for your ceiling material. As far as floors, we stayed with stained concrete floors. Be sure to use a reputable company to do your concrete staining and finish. We used some 'guys' who thought they knew... but one year later, the polyurethane started peeling. Four years later, we ended up moving all the furniture into the garage, so that a reputable, more expensive company could strip and re-stain the floor. The wax-based finish they used is wonderful and we would highly recommend that type of finish, because it's not only beautiful, but also easy to maintain.

You will have to remember, before you pour your concrete, where your bathrooms are going to go. As long as you have those firmly in place, you can build walls and set space for other rooms wherever you want to, then tear them out and reconfigure if you want to change them after several years. You don't have to shore anything up, or support anything: you just tear them out and start over.

The 60 x 60 shell that we put in, with two porches, inclusive of metal and all other materials, cost $37K. This does not include the finished interior or exterior, just the shell. A check of more recent pricing suggests you could still mimic our structure for $41K.

To finish and furnish, you can find a lot of materials on discontinued sales from other contractors. Slightly damaged goods will sell for way cheaper and demolition homes are a dream come true. Olin found replacement windows (double hung and only 2 years old) at a house that was being demolished in Brentwood. Our kitchen cabinets came out of an apartment-building remodel. If you can, you might consider befriending a contractor who can help you source this material, but sites such as Craigslist can also be very helpful.

You can also find stuff through Habitat for Humanity's Re-Store. Contractors often don't have space to store extra building materials, so they will often take discarded/replaced items down to Re-Store. We found the tile on top of our kitchen counter in a deserted warehouse storage building, and we have a lot of it still stacked on our property for future use. Besides the knowledge that this is a very "sustainable" method of finding material resources, one of the real pleasures of doing this is when you find very nice quality materials at a real bargain!

There are lots of ways to find and save money if willing to do a little extra work. As another example, the barn wood chair rail, which lines the interior of many of our rooms, was also from the Brentwood demolition house. We found 100 year old barn doors on a wall in that same home, and Olin was able to salvage them to hang on our dining room wall as a focal point of the room. (By the way, old barn wood now is gold.)

Essentially, if you find a demolition site, and can carry away what you tear down, it's yours. It's polite to ask the contractor first, but they are often only too happy to have you do this, as it can save them paying someone.

One thing to consider that is not as much of a problem for our northern neighbors is that Tennessee is a termite friendly state (another great reason to use metal as your structure!) Before bringing wood from a demolition site into the house, Olin will pressure wash any wood he plans to use inside, then dry it and inspect it for termite damage before doing so. Termites like moisture, so if you dry out the wood properly to get rid of any moisture, the termites will leave.

You can also put down coils that heat your floor before you pour your concrete. This is similar to how the Romans used to heat their villas. These can be heated via hot water or electricity, and can be very energy-efficient. You will need your thermostat to be above floor level of course!

We keep our floors clean simply with a vacuum, wet mop, and then mop 'n glow polish, which only needs to be applied once a month.

As we had a smaller space inside, we knew we needed more usable outdoor space. In the Tennessee summer, the sun can be strong very early and remain so well into the evening, so we decided to build two porches, one east and one west, and will typically use the one with the most shade at that time of day, especially when we run our classes. Depending on weather, and temperature, we may also want to be either sheltered from, or exposed to, the light and weather going on outside.

Each porch is 12 x 60 feet, and can be enclosed. For the latter, we used temporary placed plastic mosquito curtains, just like the heavy-duty 20mm ones you see at restaurants. You can get different colored ribbons on the bottom, and attach them with snaps of Velcro. Because the resulting enclosure is very easy to heat and maintain, we can have a party outside even during the winter!

We have 1400 sq. ft. of finished space downstairs, and our loft upstairs is also usable, set up as an apartment, and is about 600 sq. ft. We have almost 1500 sq. ft. of porches (1440 exactly). If using our design, you can of course use any materials you want to, and don't have to use metal, but metal makes sense from both a structural and sustainable standpoint. (You can even use metal garage doors for walls, as these lift up and close as weather conditions dictate).

In most jurisdictions, you do not have to have a contractor: you can build your house yourself. The problem you may run into, if you do this, is finding reliable subcontractors to come out to your job. (A good sub may have a lot of work with a particular contractor, and if, for example, he has 10 jobs going on with his contractor, vs. only your single job, he will put his priority where he gets the most business).

Other Building Options:

As we've indicated, there are almost unlimited ways to build your house. Below are some of the ones we feel are creative, as well as growing in popularity in various parts of the country.

Straw Bale Houses:

These are exactly what they sound like: you stack straw bales up and put a roof on them! Leigh says its "like stucco, but not quite: you put it on the straw, and it makes a seal for the walls and roof." The straw is treated to eliminate insects, but the bales need to be kept dry to prevent their return. These houses are usually more common in highly arid conditions (AZ, NM, etc.), and not in TN, with our thunderstorms and humidity. We suspect these structures wouldn't even pass as dwellings in TN, especially in Williamson Co., but they could make interesting sheds or workshops.

Tiny Houses:

You may have heard of the tiny house movement, which is growing in popularity, especially as a way for contract workers to live in a place for a fixed, finite length of time. The big question you'd want to ask yourself is: "Could I live in that?" For ourselves, we couldn't, they could be guesthouse, or B&B options. Tiny houses are not cheap; the cheapest one we could find in Nashville cost $49K.

Shipping Containers:

We seriously looked at these, as they are also metal. The containers come in different sizes, usually 40 feet long, and 8-10 feet wide. They are made of solid steel, and can accommodate wood floors. You could stack them cross ways and elevate/stack as you went higher. We saw some really nice models, having bedrooms with glass walls, as an example. You can place them around metal studs, run your wires, blow your insulation, and you're done. You can do a modular build, adding them one at a time (www.trueactivist.com). You can find these on Craigslist, for as little as $2-4K.

Containers are considered moveable, so you probably wouldn't have to worry about setback lines, in terms of placement, etc. They may be more susceptible to tornado damage than a more fixed type of house.

In Williamson County, you can't put new trailer homes on a property; ones you see have already been grandfathered in. Also in Williamson, for people to use a temporary structure as a retreat, hotel or B&B, you need to seek the proper permits and licenses, for tax purposes. You would similarly want to check your local codes before investing in any non-traditional buildings.

Water and Sewage and Lights, oh my!

As we mentioned earlier, out in the country, your soil, rock and perc (septic) tests are very important. When you go out to buy a piece of property, the number one thing you need to ensure is that it "percs," and how big of a septic area you will need. Perc is short for "percolates" (just as in the old way of making coffee), and is a measure of how quickly the soil will absorb moisture.

The perc testers will go out and dig a hole, fill it full of water, and then time how long it takes to drain. In Tennessee, there is a lot of clay-based soil, so perk times can be pretty slow.

We have two perc sites on our land. One is right where the garden is; the other one is up behind the house. Both of them have an A and B site, which are your primary and secondary discharge areas. In case one of them fails, each has a fall back. You may recall we originally intended to put a second building on the property, so we would have had to use both perc sites. Your perc site determines how many bedrooms (2 people per bedroom) you can have per septic system. Our perc sites have 3 and 2 bedroom (respectively) approvals from the county.

The siting of your septic tank will determine where you situate your house. You also need to know the local setback rules. "Setbacks" and setback lines dictate how many feet away from the property line you have to be before you can build your structure. For whatever reason, our property has a 100-foot setback line on three sides, while the one at the back where our woods are only has a 50-foot setback. If you do want to build in front of your setback line, you'll have to get a zoning variance, etc.

This is why you'll often see in housing subdivisions, new houses that are only a few feet apart, as they may only have a five foot setback line, which, apart from the land area to square footage rule of thumb, the builder may have negotiated in order to compress more houses closely together, and increase revenues.

Other important questions to ask concern the availability of water and electricity. Most people will say, "Well yeah, it's out there on the road." As long as you can get out to the road, it's not an issue. Running electricity lines can be especially tricky. If there's a pole sitting in your neighbor's yard, that you want to tie into, you have to get a written easement so the power company can drive out there onto their property. You wouldn't believe the people that will say no. Olin built a house in 1994 where he had this exact issue and he ended up going to George Jones (yes the famous country music artist and his neighbor), and asked him for his help, and George signed it. Which is how Olin got to know George Jones!

These are the kind of things you have to keep in the back of your mind when looking at a prospective property, which is another reason we stress the importance of neighbor relations.

As we mentioned in the introduction, a sustainable farm attempts to be energy-efficient. So what about alternative power sources?

We did look long and hard at these. You do have to look at the pros and cons and short and long term costs of everything. We looked at solar and wind in particular.

Let's start with solar. We met a solar salesman at the Living Green Conference at the factory in Franklin. He came out and gave us an estimate. Just to put in a basic system, barely enough to power the house, was going to be $60K! Worse, it would have taken up about half the back yard. This was about 5-6 years ago. We started doing the math, factoring in the longevity of the panels, which are rated as having a 20-year life, which basically means they have a 15-year life until you replace them. You also have to keep them very clean. If you don't keep them very clean, they won't work well.

As for the wind in our area, even to get a constant 10 mph wind, you have to be about 200 feet in the air. So now you are raising a 20 story pole (that is probably not going to please your neighbors), and you are still talking $60-$100K just to get started.

You also have to make sure that your specific local power company is going to give you credit for the power that you are not using, or for the power that you are trying to sell back to them. They wouldn't even be able to access that without the line (for which you may need to beg your neighbors), which is kind of why you would be looking at all this in the first place, (because you didn't want to have to go and beg your neighbors).

So although green energy sounds really good, especially, because of its fit with the sustainability model, when we started running the numbers for our property, it didn't really make sense. We calculated it would take 30 years for us to see a return on our investment, and that long of a return period just didn't make economic sense for us.

So what about Natural Gas? A lot of farms use propane. We use propane for our water heater, and could use it for a stove, but we have heard from other farms that it is very expensive to use for a heating/cooling system.

We would like to use our local natural gas company, but it can cost a lot of money to run a gas line in from the road. We live 2600 feet off the road and at $20 a foot that comes to $52,000, which in anybody's dictionary is real money.

Connectivity:

You almost can't exist today without Internet connectivity, and sustainable farming in particular works partly because of the small enterprise's ability to leverage modern digital technology to compete with larger farm businesses. We looked at getting Comcast. This was going to cost $9K, just for them to run the wire, and Comcast wouldn't let us run the wire ourselves. We did have Direct TV for years (satellite), but it became so expensive that we became "cable cutters" and dropped it. It was a joy to save $120 a month to just watch TV! We bought an Antenna (Home Depot and Lowes carries them) and a Smart TV, and connected both to the already existing cable from Direct TV. We are able to WIFI stream Netflix and other movie apps directly on the Smart TV. Instead of $120 per month, we now pay $8.75 for Netflix. We are confident that technology will continue to improve and provide even more affordable options.

We use DSL for our Internet access. Comcast's internet speed is way faster than what you can get with DSL, but in our experience, and that of many of our friends, almost everything else is worse, including and especially customer service. On the other hand, using DSL on a Monday morning here: good luck getting online!

4. WHY ARE YOU DOING THIS?

You may find it odd that we put this section so far into the book, and of course there would be good reasons for putting it earlier. But the plain truth is, we didn't figure out our "why" until a couple of years after we'd taken the plunge. You may find, as we did, that what you originally envision you'll be doing when you start your farm, may end up being quite different than that vision a couple of years in. Circumstances that you can't foresee, changes in your understanding of the challenges and opportunities that you are facing, and perhaps even changes in your understanding of yourself, may all contribute to not having a fixed mission for some time.

In addition, the property you buy, the house you live in, and the farm buildings you end up having may all limit or expand your potential to do certain things, closing some doors you were certain you wanted to walk through, while opening others you had no idea even existed.

So we would suggest that while it will be helpful to have at least some ideas, or even a business plan, when you first start out (if for no other reason than convincing a reluctant spouse), we'd also suggest not writing these early plans in stone, and to remain open to other paths which may present themselves as you embrace farm living.

So ask yourself at first, and then continuously: What is your mission? Why are you doing this? What do you hope to achieve?

Our mission now is to grow healthy food through sustainable

farm practices, and to teach others how to do the same. This is obviously not the mission we had when we thought we'd be opening a B&B!

How you can find your passion:

One thing we should share is that we have followed the work of Dan Miller very closely. We were in fact already reading Dan's work before we realized he was our neighbor. We discovered this about Dan because we received a big truckload of author copies of his book, *48 Days to the Work You Love*, on our porch one day completely by "accident." Now I don't want to get all Twilight Zone on you, especially if you are not consciously a person of faith, but for us what happened that day was no accident, but rather a way forward for us to find the true "why" for our farm.

I'd strongly recommend that anyone looking to reignite their passion, or to discover it in the first place, should read *48 Days to the Work You Love*, and see if it might not be of some help to you as well.

Another, big, huge, key is to not be scared, and to just "sort of go with it." For example, when we moved into Stoney Creek, our upstairs was not finished, but we moved in anyway, and we worked on the upstairs for the next two years. The shop was added a little bit here and there, largely in Olin's spare time, from things produced in his workshop. Olin built his workshop just outside the house, using, in true sustainable fashion, material that was roughly 90% recycled.

Here are some things you might want to consider when thinking about what your farm passion might be. It's not by any means an exhaustive list, but it might push a button deep inside that you didn't know you had, or it might simply get you thinking in creative ways about other, completely different opportunities unique to you:

If your passion is animals, you might want to think about meat production (cows, sheep, goats) dairy production (cows, goats), eggs (chickens, exotic birds). Or perhaps you'd like to raise something like alpacas, or even breed dogs with a kennel operation, etc.

Maybe your passion is in growing things. In that case, there is an incredible variety of vegetables, fruit, berries, or flowers that you could grow. You could start a nursery; you could raise special cash crops in local demand (hemp and hops in Tennessee for example). There are a ton of possibilities. One of our recent conference attendees had a passion for beer, so if he wanted to imitate our model, he could raise hops for the breweries, and also have a small personal beer output, so that people could come to learn and understand the whole process of brewing, just as an example.

Perhaps you might have a passion for bees, and the dwindling bee populations potentially affected by GMO crops, so you might want to have hives that have access to non-GMO crops, and sell honey, and other bee products.

An interesting local example is "Basil and Bergamot," a farm that grows unique flowers. People will buy old –fashioned, unique flowers for weddings and other events, so they have captured a unique niche in the flower market. A flower or garden plant nursery would qualify as a farm too, although the thing about nurseries is: If you start selling plants to the public, you will need to be regulated, inspected, etc. And the bigger you are, the more this happens.

Generally speaking, the smaller your operation, the less you'll have to be inspected, the larger you are the more inspection you face, to protect the public.

It's perhaps useful to note that farm size is measured by quantity sold (not land acreage or revenue). We sell about 3 doz. eggs a week. (156 dozen a year) and can house 3,000 hens without being inspected by USDA. But if you get above that, you will have to be inspected. In addition, if you sell to a grocery store or to a market or a farmer's market, then you must have the eggs inspected, for public health reasons.

How do you know/find out what the limits are on small-scale sales that will not reach the threshold for inspection by USDA? Your state Agriculture Extension website will have this information, and it is freely available.

We don't want to put a damper on anybody's dreams, but inspection and regulation, as well as zoning, will definitely determine the size and nature of your operation. As a for instance, we were going to sell pickles, as we have a famous family recipe that people just love, which I call 'Mama's Candy Pickles'. As it turns out, pickles have to be made in a commercial kitchen, which is not a home kitchen, but rather a food-safe kitchen operating as a separate space, with a closed door, special venting, etc.

Some foods that you sell are ok to make in a home kitchen, but if you sell them off-site (like at a farmer's market) you will need to affix a label that says: "Made in a home kitchen that was not inspected." The online sales of foodstuffs run into the same regulations.

You need to be aware of what the regulations are around the production of any food items you wish to sell to the public. Typically, the acidity and sugar content of the food you make will determine the level of regulation it requires. Jams and jellies are ok: pickles are not.

Pickles have all these regulations: so do salsa, pepper sauces, hot sauces, etc. You can't just sell pickles. You CAN sell any baked goods item made in your kitchen no problem, and you can sell any jam or jelly too. But if you want to sell a pickle, you have to have a food safety sink (three compartment sink, like a restaurant).

You can't have a pet in your kitchen, or anywhere in your house if you want to be able to tout a food safe kitchen. You have to place certain labels on the product as well: "Made in a non-inspected kitchen."

Such regulations are important for protecting the health of the public. There are horror stories of people getting killed from eating bad food product that came in jars. One of the stories I heard at a local food safety seminar was about the Hein family. Delphine and Edward threw a dinner party 80 years ago at their farm in ND. Delphine served a salad with peas sprinkled from her own home canned pantry. Within days, 13 people fell ill and died, including the Heins and three of their 6 children. Authorities determined that the home-canned peas were to blame by toxins produced from Clostridium botulinum bacteria, which causes botulism poisoning.

All this being said, if you really want to make your family's home-made hot sauce, and do not have a food-safe commercial kitchen, you can often find rental space for these not too far from where you live. We have one of these in Franklin, TN, for example. You simply rent the space for the time you need.

Another option is to get someone to produce it for you and give them a cut of the profits.

For instance, when you visit a pumpkin patch farm, e.g., other people have likely produced the farm-branded jams and jellies you buy there. There are people (2 or 3 companies) who will do this for you, for your jelly, molasses, etc., and put your label on it. But it's their recipe. Some will make your recipe to your specs. But because you will typically ask for a much shorter production than they normally do, you will pay proportionally much more per item, and will therefore make a very low margin (a few cents) from going that route. When a third party does it for you using their recipe they may sell it to you for, say, $3, and if you sell it to the public for $5, your margins will be much higher.

It all depends on which way you want to go, and what really lights your fire. If you want to take your own recipe to the top, you can do a test market, before you go to the expense of getting somebody to produce it for you on a large scale.

But did we mention you could buy somebody else's stuff and pop your label on it?

How about growing fruit trees?

Well, we didn't do our research properly, so when we first came to the farm, we thought: (Imagine your best Valley Girl voice) "Oh, like, let's put in Apple Trees!" As it turns out, Stoney Creek Farm has got to be one of the worst properties in the world to grow any kind of fruit tree.

We have killed four peach trees so far. Cedar rust takes over every year on the apple crop. Another problem is squirrels. We've put traps out for squirrels, but it doesn't matter: they are going to get your apples. Squirrels in TN are very smart. This might sound a little redneck, but our rodents are geniuses.

We've gone through all this heartache for one simple reason: we just did not do our research, so our takeaway message is: do your research, and don't do like we did.

Just so you know, cedar trees can spread a detrimental fungus to apple trees. *Gynnosporangium juniperi-virginianae* is a plant pathogen that causes "cedar-apple rust". It is a disfiguring and often destructive disease of both the apples and cedars. This disease comes from having cedar trees in the vicinity, and you would have to spray them liberally every week, and then that still might not work. But we are not big fans of spraying: we don't like doing that, partly because it's time consuming and expensive, and partly because of our general sustainable (that word again) philosophy of trying to leave as small a chemical footprint as we can. So, we just gave up on the fruit trees. We invested about $300 for the two little orchards. It would be better to have more blueberries or blackberries, as these are not affected by cedar rust, so we are expanding those fruits. Olin wants fruit trees so badly, every time one of them dies, he puts a new one in its place, and Leigh doesn't say a word. Just do your research.

Navigating Rules and Crowds to Find Something Unique:

Maybe you've thought about developing an Agritourism farm. At the risk of sounding mean: do you have a passion for kids coming in and tearing up your farm? If you do, then you have to do one of these, because that's exactly what happens. If not, then maybe this type of farm business isn't right for you.

If you are a baker, you can sell almost any kind of baked goods any time, as long as you are not trying to do it in huge volumes. These are not subject to the strict regulations on pickles. You don't even have to put that they are not from a food-safe kitchen on the label. You can sell them at yard sales, farmer's markets, church functions, etc.

There are no regulations on soap either. But remember: anything that you would can or jar other than jams or jellies, and I do mean anything: tomatoes, soups, salsas, anything, you will need to prepare them in a food safe kitchen before you can sell any of that.

Do you like to teach? Ta Da! That is what we do. That is what we discovered, after some trial and error, is where we really shine, and is what we love to do. So, we are a teaching farm. That's our goal, our passion, and our mission. When we figured that out, we were two years into this. That means, two years into opening up the farm to the public. We'd already been five years playing around with the fruit trees, goats and chickens, finally got serious, most likely because our CPA made sure we knew that we could be tagged as a 'hobby farm', instead of a real working farm. Hobby farms are not allowed to take deductions and depreciation on taxes. Our goal was to be a real working farm and make a difference in people's lives…so we needed to actually make money or be classified as a non-profit. After researching non-profit requirements (having a board, paperwork, etc.), our choice was to make money on the operation.

So we began to look around at other farms to see what they were doing. Olin has family in Mississippi (Mitchell Farm), who operates a big pumpkin patch every fall. Over 30,000 people go there every year to buy their fall pumpkins and enjoy fun activities like farm animals, tiny town, gem-mining and tractor rides, to name a few. To learn more about what they do, see http://www.mitchellfarms-ms.com.

There are farms near ours that do a pumpkin patch and corn mazes. We don't want to do a pumpkin patch here, because we do not want to compete with our sister farms and quite frankly, do not want 10 - 30,000 kids trampling our small farm of 15 acres. We also had no desire to manage 15 – 20 employees for an 8-week period, having to deal with human resource issues, etc. Fortunately for us, it wasn't our passion anyway.

Lucky Ladd farms in Murfreesboro started a petting zoo. They do an outstanding job and offer a ton of activities for the kids. They have a huge playground, pumpkin launcher, slides and too much more to mention. They have miniature donkeys the kids can ride when they are there: it's a really neat place.

Once we looked at what other farms were offering in the area, we started to think about what could be a unique offering in this area, and that's where Olin came up with idea of renting garden plots. Nobody else was doing it; nobody else has a U-Pick Garden in this area, either. Olin came up with the garden plot rental idea (you rent the plot, and grow your own stuff). Leigh came up with the U-Pick Garden idea (we grow the stuff, and you buy it). Leigh's uncle, Jerry Parker, told her (he's a retired County Ag Extension agent), "You just need to have a vegetable stand, or go to a farmer's market and do that." And you know, I just really didn't want to do that, and I battled with the idea, and we finally did the mission statement thing, and realized it didn't fit the mission statement of teaching people how to live sustainably. But the U-Pick is a variation on that idea, and it does fit the mission.

We now have 15 plots (and growing), priced at $75 - 125/growing season (April – October). This income stream covers our liability insurance, etc., and translates into about $1500 worth of revenue, which covers us for the Greenbelt classification under the Tax Code.

When we first came up with the idea, we mapped out the property into grids. We thought of having several hundred grids, but crowd control and other issues (water expense, e.g.) put a stop to this plan. We currently use rainwater capture for the gardeners to water their rental plots, but we would not be able to provide that much rainwater for a host of people.

Many of the finer points for our mission evolved over time, as new information came to light. A lot of it was a process of elimination: trying and discarding ventures that were, somehow, "not us." If you are in a bigger hurry than we were, it would be best if you could avoid going down as many blind alleys as we did, and that idea contributed to the rationale for this book.

Because we had the luxury of being able to be in trial and error mode for a few years, the big determinants for us when we thought of trying out a new idea were: if it wasn't going to cost a lot, and we didn't have much to lose if it didn't work out, we would go for it. Sometimes it would work, more often it didn't, but now we have a much better understanding about what we want to do, what we can do, and what we are allowed to do than when we started.

There are definitely ways to make money without spending a lot of money. But you'll always need to spend at least a little bit of money in order to make money (there is no way around that). Olin's mantra is: Just Do Something, even if it's wrong, because you will learn a lot from doing it, and you may come up with a better idea for doing it, or a different idea that really takes off.

So you can't be too stubborn, or too negative. Some people are very afraid of change: Olin says he used to be that way. Now, the prospect of change is not an issue for him. If things aren't changing, you probably aren't doing something right.

Another idea might be to put in a labyrinth. This is easy to do, and provides a walking meditation space. You can ask for a donation ($2?) Or provide free admission if someone takes a class/buys something at your store, etc. Walking the labyrinth has a very strong history in the Christian faith, but is non-denominational and a powerful prayer/meditation/problem-solving technique. You can also get listed on the national "labyrinth site" registry, which would help get your place, quite literally, on the map.

Ask yourself, if there is a working business model, outside of your local area, perhaps in another state, that no one near you is doing, that fits your passion?

We researched Polyface Farms owned by Joel Salatin. He raises all types of naturally grown meat, and is a champion of sustainable farming. We visited him in Virginia in 2014, to see his operation and learn from his methods. Needless to say, we were very impressed. He produces the exact amount of chickens where you don't have to be USDA inspected. He processes that many chickens a year, and no more. He has it down to a science, and to us, he just has a lot of good sense. We ultimately decided that we didn't want to do meat. It's pretty messy for our taste (and sad as well, to be honest). But what we did learn from Joel was how to pay for help without breaking the bank. Because you will not find farm labor "on the cheap." So we offer volunteer positions here (akin to internships) where you look for people who want to learn about what you do. We have one main intern, who has been with me more than two years, one who is beginning her second year, and two other interns that help with the farm.

In addition to being less expensive, this model helps you to find people who are willing to do things your way. Someone with experience may have preconceived ideas about how they want to do things. This means a) you should have at least a pretty good knowledge of what good practices are, and b) also be willing to invest some time in teaching someone those practices, because that is the contract you are basically making with someone who is coming to work with you on this volunteer basis.

In appreciation for their help our volunteers can attend our seminars, mostly for free. If I have a speaker, I do ask they contribute the speaker fee. They get free sourdough starter, they get free kefir grains, etc. For anything that has to do with running the farm, they have to help us for 8 hours a week, and then they get free veggies/eggs/herbs and more. All of our interns are treated like our family. That's how you get help without breaking the bank.

As another example, if you decide your passion is fitness, then ask, what fits with that? Perhaps a fitness/obstacle course works with that. Grass-fed beef works with that. Herbs and non-cow dairy may also be a draw. Dog breeding could be a fit as an agriculture activity, especially if, as an example, you picked a breed like the Great Pyrenees (a protection dog for goats). Even dog health can be a specialty for your farm, as many dogs are now becoming obese. I grow one customer's organic plants for her in our greenhouse, whose farm is called Borderline farms. She has an agility training facility for dogs and also trains diabetic alert dogs. (A diabetic alert dog will come and alert you or a family member if your insulin/glucose levels get out of whack. You could raise Seeing Eye dogs, or hearing ear dogs.

We mentioned that the U-Pick Garden is part of our mission. But to be clear, the u-pick is the draw that gets people to come and visit us, and we do it on a very small scale as a result, hoping that these visitors will be encouraged to return to one of our classes and learn about sustainable living.

Mitchell Farms in Collins, MS was an example of a big, u-pick operation. They used to have a 100-acre U-Pick Garden (we have 2 acres!), and people would come from miles around to go there. They sold hundreds of pounds of butterbeans, peas, etc. and they were traditional farmers.

This was all very hard work, and as a few of the family members became older they turned it into an Agritourism farm, where they do a pumpkin patch every year, as mentioned earlier. This means their main source of income for the whole year goes on for 8 weeks. They charge $10 a ticket (just to come in), and they have thousands of people who visit during that period, so you can do the math.

At the same time, you should realize: operations at that scale are big business. It sounds attractive from the revenue stream, but the organizational coordination required to run an operation of that size is huge. They carry big liability insurance, because every year, someone may have an accident or incident that could be a liability to the farm. They are very proactive about safety for visitors, but sometimes it's impossible to control all things of this nature.

We don't want to run something that demanding: Leigh is retired, from big business and wants to do something that's meaningful to her in a different way. She wants to enjoy what she does. Leigh retired at 53 from the corporate world. She was travelling 7 states, no passion left, making lots of money, but wasn't happy, and that life just wasn't worth it anymore.

Olin retired at the end of 2017 when he sold his share of the partnership to two of the other partners. Although he still consults with Development and Property Management companies, he is now able to spend a lot more time at the farm, making a difference in the community.

Another part of sustainable living was becoming debt free, and de-cluttering our life of irrelevant material possessions. We generally adhere to the techniques and behaviors espoused by Dave Ramsey, the author of Financial Peace and The Total Money Makeover. We have followed the principles laid out in his books, and, through careful planning and very disciplined budgeting, we can say that they do work. We only pay cash for cars. We have a budget that we live on, which forces us to save. We can't draw out of our 401k and other retirement funds until we are 59 ½, (and Leigh quit at 53), so we need and want to be disciplined about our spending.

We have no debt on our property, and love to share the fact that the grass feels different when you walk on your bare feet on ground you've paid off. Twelve years ago, we got rid of our credit cards. Simplifying your life is about freedom, and not having debt is unbelievably freeing. We lived on very little money for a couple of years while still making good money, became debt free FIRST, then felt financially able to make the transition to the farm.

To embrace sustainable concepts, we'd also suggest following a minimalist mindset. A lot of us are chasing "stuff." As I've mentioned before, when we bought this property, Olin brought me here kicking and screaming. Part of this was due to my ongoing addiction to "stuff." But people are misguided to put all their hopes and dreams into stuff, so I became a minimalist. We've had larger houses, nicer décor, and a lot more "stuff" in the past, but it was not as meaningful as our home is today. We'd say: hang and/or display the stuff in your house that has some kind of family meaning to you.

Another thing to try is to simplify your wardrobe. Leigh is aspiring to have what she calls an encapsulated wardrobe. She is in the process of pairing down her wardrobe to have 8 outfits for each season; mixing and matching the pieces, which simplifies the whole process of building a wardrobe and choosing your daily clothing. It's very freeing to have this kind of mindset.

We also stopped eating out as much, especially fast food. You save a ton of money by doing this. We invested in maintenance-free housing. Olin takes the pressure washer and washes the house once a year. He also does repurposing and recycling of other discarded materials, wood pieces especially, that's his forte.

We bought furniture that wears well, and lasts a long time.

We'd also suggest surrounding yourself with people of like values. If you want to be out of debt, don't hang with people with a lot of debt, and/or who put a lot of value on having a lot of stuff. Don't keep up with the Joneses. Fill your life with stories to tell, not stuff to show.

Simplifying your life will help you reach your goals faster (not spending it on shoes, etc.) Also, you don't have to worry about having the right home in the right neighborhood, and if that's what you already have, especially if you've worked really hard to get there, stepping out of that can feel scary. It can feel like you are going backwards.

Sustainability is about "Thrive not Survive." Stuff weighs you down. It's not sustainable. And if too much of your energy becomes directed towards the acquisition or preservation of your stuff, trust us, whether you realize it or not you are surviving not thriving. We aren't judgmental about people who are scared to take this leap: we do understand that a mindset change is required to give up the stuff. Leigh had a suburban house with an HOA, drove a Mercedes, she had all that "stuff," but especially after the kids were grown, it seemed as if something inside her changed. Some people cannot afford enough furniture to fill up their huge houses because they are up to their eyeballs in debt: they are house rich and cash poor.

So we came to understand that giving up stuff was not about enduring a loss; it was about giving ourselves permission to do things differently. It's about feeling privileged to have the freedom. As a culture we're addicted to the notion that achievement, and the visible trappings of achievement, equals success, and it's only now that many of us are reverting to the notion that a life of meaning, is the way to success.

Other Things to Consider in the Hunt for Your Passion:

Choose something you already find fascinating and love to talk about.

Also choose something where your life experiences add to your understanding.

Make sure it something you have a seed of a talent for. Remember, her initial resistance notwithstanding, Leigh did already know how to grow stuff. She also knew how much hard work any kind of farming, sustainable or otherwise, requires.

One thing to remember is that Google is your friend. You can find out almost anything on Google.

Make sure it's something you want to heavily invest your time and energy in for the next five years. Olin and Leigh spent a lot of time working their 'real jobs' and working on the farm. They do not recommend this, as "it like to have killed us." Initially, it may be helpful if one member of the partnership can focus on the homestead, while the other does their day job.

We looked at structuring the farm as a 501(c)(3), with non-profit status. We decided against that, as it was too complicated for us, and we especially didn't want to have a board we would have to answer to. If you go down this road, you will need to have a deep passion for the over-arching philosophy of your non-profit to do it.

We don't take any federal grant money, although we could take quite a bit. Why not? It's a conscious choice. We do not want to fall under any federal or state program requirements. Since autonomy is obviously a very big thing for us, it doesn't fit with who we are, but that may not be as much of an issue for other people. By the way, there is a lot of federal grant money available, just check with your local Agriculture Extension Agent or CPS (Crop Production Services).

Whether or not you accept a grant, there may be a lot of regulations around your business model, production, etc. Suppose you say: I want to get into producing ABC, the FIRST thing you need to do is discover the rules and regulations governing how you must do it. What the associated costs are. What the liability is, and how it could affect insurance. So if you are doing it in large part for the freedom, as we are, you would want to be careful about engaging in an activity, or government oversight, that would impact your freedom.

Test out your proposed business idea on a small scale. How does it work? Would you do it again? We've done lots of things that we've decided not to do again. Also, if it's successful, and you love it, it can take over your life.

Olin tells a story about how he worked at a farmer's market when he was young: picked watermelons, put them in the back of a truck, took them to market, sold them, turned around, picked some more, did it again. Depending on the area Farmer's Markets can be anywhere from $20 - $100 just to get a booth. So now you start doing the math:

"OK I've spent $100. I have to buy the gas to drive over there. Do I need any special transport items (refrigerated truck, ice, e.g.) Pick it, clean it, transport it, sell $100 worth just to get my fee back."

But the answer to whether it's worth it or not is different for every person. For some people it could be totally worth it to do this, depending on how much effort/time they want to put into doing it. We would rather have people come out here (spend their gas), bring their kids, turn them loose, don't have to worry about anything bad happening to them. They don't have to worry about where their produce is coming from: it's right outside! Our feedback from the people having this experience is what makes it worthwhile to us: how we are able to enrich people's lives by providing the experience.

The people pick it; we weigh it, sit on the porch, drink a bottle of water, and talk with us. This is why you have to really decide what the purpose of your farm is. Our purpose is not necessarily to find some hot item to grow and sell at a market, but to invite people out to the property for a vanishing experience that is getting harder and harder to find and duplicate. Some customers liken the experience to "Going back in time to their Grandparents' home."

Everything you do should tie into your purpose and your mission. Famer's Markets and the rest do not tie into our mission (though they might yours), because they are not teaching anybody anything, they are just selling something. Not that there's anything wrong with selling something, if that's your passion, and what the purpose and mission of your farm is, but we wanted specifically to teach others how to share in the experiences, or even just to offer it.

And that's the long, winding path we took to find our passion, and the reason for this book is to hopefully help you find yours in a little shorter time than it took us.

5. GROWING HEALTHY FOOD

Although we grew up on traditional farms, that was different from a) having a farm open to the public, and b) having a sustainable farm. We had some learning, and some unlearning, to do. We've learned the most lessons about what we should offer at Stoney Creek in the last five years.

The first year, Leigh killed 2/3 of the tomato plants by over-fertilizing them. She says: "Every year, I do something really stupid, but that's ok, because its part of the learning experience. Actually, it's probably more naïve than stupid, I make these mistakes because I don't know any better, but I learn from it. Stupid would be making the same mistakes every year and expecting different results."

It all starts with the soil:

As sustainable farmers, we understand that healthy soils translate into healthy plants (and thereby healthy people). Although plants (and people) can often grow under poor conditions a sustainable approach to farming depends on treating your soil as much more than just "dirt," and instead as the living treasure it is: a treasure that serves as the building block of the sustainable cycle from the land, to plants, and then to animals (including us), and back again.

The condition of your soil today is a result of what has happened to it in the sometimes incredibly far distant, as well as the more recent, past. Both natural (for example: erosion) and manmade (cultivation) forces have almost certainly had an effect on the nature of your soil. These effects will determine how much and when it can support plant growth, as well as what type of plants will thrive in it.

How well you take care of your soil, then, is as important a step in sustainable farming as how well you tend your plants, or how well you take care of your animals. This might seem obvious, but many beginning farmers may not understand how to properly prepare the soil on their farms before planting. But with proper testing, care, and amending (fixing any soil problems or issues), it is possible even for the beginner to have excellent, dark, loamy soil in which to grow the best crops.

Soil quality is typically evaluated on the two broad measures of texture and fertility.

Soil Texture:

Soil texture measures the size of the soil particles, and their ability to stick to each other, or cohesiveness. Soil texture may be classified as clay, sandy or loamy.

Sandy soils have very large particles. Water, air and plant roots can move freely in sandy soils, sometimes too much so. Sandy soils are just what they sound like – they are actually high in sand, and drain quickly.

At the other end of the spectrum is clay. Clay soils tend to be rich in nutrients, but retain a lot of water. Clay particles are so small, that they are tightly packed together, leaving little room for additional water, air or roots. If you've ever tried to dig in a bed of baked clay, it can seem as iron-hard as the shovel blade itself.

An easy test for soil texture is to make a ball of damp garden soil. If it breaks apart when you tap it, it's sandy. If you can press it between your thumb and finger and make a ribbon with it, it's clay.

Most soils are usually between these two extremes, and the soil considered the best for growing plants you'd want on a farm is something called a sandy loam. Loamy soils retain moisture without becoming "boggy," and they are relatively "fluffy" because they have air pockets. They are also high in nutrients. Soil should be light, and allow for air and water movement, but also have some "tilth," a gritty texture not unlike breadcrumbs, which usually occurs when there is plenty of organic matter in the soil.

A big mistake some beginners make is trying to change their soil's texture by adding sand to clay or vice versa. But this process is just a recipe for cement. So don't do it.

Soil Fertility:

Soil Fertility is a measure of how many of the essential nutrients are present in the soil, and in what quantities, combined with a measure of acidity or alkalinity (pH) that affects how available these nutrients may be to plants.

Nutrients:

The three primary nutrients used by plants are nitrogen, phosphorus and potassium.

Nitrogen is largely responsible for healthy leaf and stem growth. In the soil, certain types of bacteria help convert nitrogen into nitrates, the form of nitrogen that plants can use. Nitrogen gets washed out of soil pretty quickly, but it is possible to have an excess of nitrogen, which will cause a lot of leaf growth, at the expense of flowers and fruit.

The nutrient that is most important for root growth is phosphorous. Flowering bulbs and root crops need to have enough phosphorous to be productive.

Potassium is important for overall plant health. It keeps the plants growing and aids their immune systems. Potassium, like nitrogen, dissolves in water, and needs to be replenished from time to time.

Besides these three primary nutrients, there are several trace elements that are necessary for good plant health like: calcium, magnesium, zinc, molybdenum, etc.

Soil pH:

You can read a lot about soil pH, and its affect on plant growth. As we've said, for the non-scientists, pH measures the soil's acidity or alkalinity.

The pH scale goes from 1.0 to 14.0, with 7.0 being neutral (7 is the pH of water). The lower the number below 7, the more acidic the soil is, the higher above 7, the more alkaline. Soil pH is important because plants can only access and use the nutrients in the soil if the soil pH is within a certain range. Many plants like a pH in the low acid to neutral range (6.2 - 6.8), but that's not true for all plants.

Differences in desired soil pH is a big reason that you can't always have certain combinations of plants in the same soil bed. Rhododendrons, heathers and blueberries favor very acidic soils, and lilacs and clematis will thrive in alkaline or even chalky soil. The only foolproof way to know where your soil's pH falls is to have it tested. It's worth keeping in mind that a) it takes time to alter soil pH and b) that over time your soil will tend to revert to its original pH (which in turn will mean repeated treatment).

Soil pH is affected by factors such as rainfall and the kinds of fertilizers applied. Strategies to lower soil pH include adding lime (which is something we do on our farm). Raising soil pH often requires adding wood ashes.

Soil Testing:

Your state's Ag extension document will tell you how to collect the proper soil samples from your soil, as well as what tests they will do for a standard fee. For more detailed information see the following site for UT Agriculture Extension Service for soil testing: https://ag.tennessee.edu/spp/Pages/soiltesting.aspx

There are two ways to test the soil in TN: by acreage or per 100 feet of garden space for a garden an acre or less. We recommend that you test per 100 feet, unless you have many acres and multiple large crops.

In Tennessee, the UT Ag Extension tells us to take ten soil samples six inches deep around your garden. Place the samples in a five gallon bucket, mix it really well, then take a subsample after its mixed up, take it to your lab, and they will test it for you.

Soil tests typically do not test for nitrogen, because the levels are too volatile, although you can order an optional soil test for nitrate levels. (Nitrate testing is usually taken at the end of the growing season. High levels mean that you may not need to add nitrogen the following spring.)

Standard soil tests do provide information on the levels of phosphorus and potassium/potash in your soil. The report will typically include recommendations for improving soil fertility, and you can ask to have the recommendations focus on organic solutions.

The UT Ag Extension soil-testing document says: "[The] Plus test includes soil pH, Mehlich-1 extractable phosphorus, potassium, calcium, magnesium, zinc, manganese, iron, sodium, and boron. Fertilizer and lime recommendations are also included." The Plus test costs $15. To additionally test for organic matter costs $15; Soluble Salts $10; Sulfur $10 and Texture (USDA) $30. If your growing material is highly organic, a container media analysis is recommended. The Container Media Test is mainly useful to greenhouse growers in determining fertility of soil-less mixtures. Turnaround is typically 1 to 2 business days (for routine Basic or

Plus) and results are routinely mailed but can be e-mailed or faxed.

Test results are used to formulate research-based, cost effective lime and fertilizer recommendations specific to the type of crop or plant and yield desired. (View a soil sample test report with an explanation of recommendations.) To assist growers with their soil fertility needs, Extension county agents are available statewide to help with any management decisions related to soil test recommendations."

Don't you feel better now? Actually, it's not that complicated, and the Ag extension folks really are very helpful.

When to Test Your Soil:

For perennial crops - orchards, pasture, Christmas trees, alfalfa, grass seed, and so on, you should test your soil before planting (preferably at least several months before), so that you have time to lime the soil and have it mix with the existing soil before planting your crop. Limestone reacts slowly with the soil, so it's important when adding lime to your soil that you leave enough lead-time before planting.

For annual crops, such as vegetables, test your soil every spring before planting for the season.

Amending Your Soil:

Your soil report will help you determine if you need to repair (amend, in farm-speak) any soil issues. Once you know what kind of soil you have, and if it has any pH issues or nutrient deficiencies, you can begin amending it.

Adjusting pH:

Changing pH can be more complex than it seems at first. It's important to understand that pH changes slowly so give it time, and retest your soil. You might also want to think about choosing crops that work with your existing soil pH. For acidic soil, you can add lime. This year, for instance, we had to add 1500 lbs. of lime pellets.

For a soil that's too alkaline, you can add sulphur or peat moss to make it more acidic.

Adding Organic Material or Compost:

Like soil pH, organic matter gets a lot of press. Organic matter is dead plant or animal material. There is always some organic matter in your soil, but often not enough for a plant's needs. Decaying organic matter, or humus, will help give your soil the tilth factor we talked about earlier. It helps sandy soil by retaining water that would otherwise wash away, and it improves clay soil by making it looser, so that air, water and roots can penetrate. In all soils, organic matter encourages beneficial microbial activity and provides some nutritional benefits.

Increasing the amount of organic matter is probably one of the most important things you can do to improve your soil, no matter what its current type. Compost, animal manure, grass clippings, leaf mold, and green manures (cover crops) are all great organic matter to add. At least three inches of organic matter spread over the surface to be planted should be added - and four to six is better.

Compost is a rich source of organic matter for growing food. Not only does composting add soil nutrients, but it also improves the structure of the soil, which enhances the process of moving moisture and nutrients from the soil into the growing plants.

To initiate compost, you can buy something, like a compost barrel, from Home Depot or Lowe's (careful! These get heavy!!), or you can build with wooden pallets, Put a pallet on bottom, then three pallets on the sides, use 2x4's in the front as slats. To start your pile, put a little hay on the bottom, with equal parts topsoil. Dump in veggie scraps etc. on an ongoing basis, and watch it become compost!

Your pile will need to be kept moist, so cover it when not in use: an old lawn tarp can be good for this. Then, the more you turn it the better: if you turn it every day, you might get compost within about four weeks.

If you don't even want to go to that trouble, you can even just use fence wire spread in a corner.

Inside the pile, microbial activity makes it start heating, which is why you turn it. You can use leaves (great for composting), but not grass clippings (you don't want to add weeds, and grass has seeds that will remain in it.) Although these will take longer than leaves, you can also use bark or tree mulch. But don't use tree limbs; you want stuff that will break down. In general, be careful what you put in it so that it doesn't have unwanted seeds. With tomatoes you want to be careful you haven't add any plants that had a disease.

Chicken waste can take a long time (months) to become compost due to its high ammonia content. Cow and horse dung takes much less time. If you use horse dung, a lot of farmers say that the weed seeds are still present, so ruminators are better because they chew and chew and chew their food (as we'll learn later in this book). It's better to use goat or cow manure than horse.

Compost is not that big a deal, although you can make it as complicated as you want. Trust us, if you are running a farm you won't have the time to do that, so just keep it simple.

Coffee grounds are good in compost, and so are eggshells, (but not eggs, or meat or other animal protein sources.) You want to attract earthworms, etc., so you'll want to leave the bottom of your pile open so earthworms can get in there. If you haven't done that, then throw some earthworms in there to start things off. Worm castings are very rich, so that really helps the compost pile. You can dig worms up in your garden, get them from a bait shop, or even buy composting worms. One person we know even has a compost worm farm in his garage!

In Franklin, TN, we have a terrific compost site run by the city.

The city picks up limbs and leaves during the fall, and uses all of it for compost. They allow anyone to buy a yard (quite a bit) of compost for about $20. You might want to investigate your own city or county for this same service. You can visit Franklin's website at this URL:

http://www.franklin-gov.com/government/streets/purchase-compost

Plant Cover Crops

Cover crops, also called green manures or living mulch, are a great way to improve soil aeration and texture, add nitrogen, and support and encourage microorganisms and worms.

They are versatile plants that are grown to suppress weeds, help build and improve the long-term sustainability of your soil, and control diseases and pests. They can add nitrogen to your soil, and build fertility without using chemical fertilizer. You can plant them in between rows of other crops to help suppress weeds, while also building fertility. They often have taproots that help break up compacted soils and improve their structures. They help control erosion, holding onto valuable, rich topsoil in between plantings. They help hold soil moisture. And they can even build disease resistance in other crops

It's important to choose the proper cover crop for the season - for example, winter rye is a fall crop, while buckwheat is sensitive to frost. Grains such as oats or rye tend to add lots of organic matter to the soil, while legumes such as field peas or hairy vetch fix nitrogen. Sometimes, farmers combine several cover crops, such as a field peas/oats mix - to gain the benefits of each type of plant. Different cover crops provide different benefits, suit your climate better or worse than others, and match your needs best at a certain time. You might plant red clover between rows of vegetable crops to control weeds, but plant buckwheat in a field that is fallow for a season, to build fertility and improve the soil's structure. In the fall, you may want to plant winter rye or vetch, but in the spring, plant sorghum.

Here are some cover crop ideas, many of which you can find discussed online as well:

Rye: Winter rye, or cereal rye, is a great cover crop to plant in the fall or early winter. It loosens compacted soil and suppresses weeds too. It also fixes excess nitrogen in the soil.

Buckwheat: Buckwheat grows very quickly, and makes a great ground cover that prevents erosion and suppresses weeds. Because of its fast-growing nature, it can be planted among other crops, and it can be planted through late summer.

Clovers: Crimson clover, red clover, and white Dutch clover are all used as cover crops. Clovers fix nitrogen in the soil and are great for improving your soil's fertility. Yellow clover is ideal for improving soil structure. Medium red clover has an array of benefits and is often used by small farmers to plant between vegetable rows.

Crimson clover is one of our favorite covers. In October, we plant crimson cover, let it cover our plot over the winter, then before we plant again, we till it in and plant in that plot a few weeks later

Sorghum (or Sudangrass) is a hybrid crop that grows quickly while putting down an extensive root structure. Like many other cover crops, it too can be used to prevent erosion and suppress weeds. It also adds biomass to the soil since it grows so tall.

Hairy Vetch is a cover crop that's very winter-hardy, and perfect for northern climates. We don't use it much in warm Tennessee It also adds a lot of nitrogen to the soil, and if allowed to grow over the winter into May, it can seriously improve soil fertility.

Adjusting nutrient levels:

Often, adding organic matter and giving it time will be enough to balance out the nutrient profile of your soil. But if your soil test showed great imbalances, you might need to directly add nutrients to your soil. You can increase phosphorous levels by adding blood meal, and calcium via bone meal, while most potassium deficiencies can be fixed by adding kelp or greensand.

Remember, if you want to call your farm "organic" you will need to do specific soil amendments as mandated by your state Ag Dept. There are very specific amendments required if you want to label yourself as an "organic" farmer. Which brings us to (fanfare, please):

A Word About Fertilizers:

As we've mentioned, "sustainable" and "organic" are not the same thing, and there is good reason to question the long-term sustainability of chemical fertilizers, which may cause a lot of damage to the environment, not only due to water runoff, but also due to the part they play in climate change.

In terms of economic sustainability, a soil-building program based on organic material probably makes much more sense than the direct addition of chemical fertilizers, especially as the costs of nitrogen fertilizer are rising dramatically

An inexpensive investment in soil testing can help sustainable farmers make the long-term changes that promote continued soil health without relying on the problematic quick-fix that chemical fertilizers promise.

In the absence of any soil amendments, your plot/field should lie fallow every few years (the bible says every 7) but this isn't always feasible for a small farmer. It's always a good idea to rotate your crops, (e.g. plant tomatoes where you had corn last year).

The Health Benefits of Gardening:

There are several scientific studies, which suggest measurable health benefits may be associated with gardening, and growing plants outdoors. Though these studies are small, these benefits may include:

1. Stress-relief and Increased Self Esteem

2. Improvement in Heart Health and Stroke Risk Reduction

3. Increased Hand Strength and Dexterity

4. Improved Brain Health and Reduced Risk for Alzheimer's disease

5. Improved Immune System Strength

6. Improved Scores on Depression and other Mental Health

Even without these scientifically suggested benefits, we are big fans of gardening, because of the way we've seen people embrace the opportunity to do it. As we've mentioned, we offer both u-pick, and rental options for the public to visit our farm

In our U-Pick Garden we grow a wide variety of vegetables, from tomatoes, to beans, to squash, corn, cucumbers, lettuce, spinach and kale, as well as a variety of peppers and berries.

After many years of experimentation concerning "what to grow", we have settled comfortably with the bulk of our plantings/seeds being tomatoes (250 plants), green beans (approx. 1/8 acre), purple-hull peas (approx. 1/8 acre), corn (½ acre). We cultivate approximately 1 acre in the U-Pick Garden, so the rest of the produce fills in what's left.

We grow the most popular veggies and fruit that are in demand in our area. All of the veggies have pests, but the fruit (blackberries, blueberries, grapes) is only bothered by Japanese Beetles (which we pick off by hand because none of the organic treatments work).

Buckwheat and Cosmos are the best plants for attracting beneficial insects (which we'll talk about later on) because their flowers are so open, and the pollen is easy for the insects to get to. We also grow marigolds and certain herbs among the plants. Marigolds deter certain insects and deer, which although cute, can be a real nuisance to our crop yields. Certain herbs are companion plants to produce and help deter insects (confuses their smell)...such as Basil and Tomatoes. Basil not only helps deter certain pests, but also make the tomatoes taste better.

We don't grow English peas, pole beans, asparagus, and certain varieties of heirloom tomatoes (as these are too susceptible to disease). The peas and pole beans force us to build stakes for them to climb... we find this to be too much effort and expense, since we already spend so much on staking 250 tomato plants.

In the rental gardens, EVERYBODY grows...Tomatoes. A lot of people also grow kale and lettuce. We also see a wide variety of peppers, herbs, flowers (sunflowers, zinnias and marigolds), cantaloupe, watermelon, sweet potatoes, red potatoes, cucumbers, sweet peas, green beans, corn, and all varieties of herbs, squash, and zucchini. For three years we had a Japanese family who grew several Japanese vegetables (Japanese cucumbers and eggplant, for example). Yoshi and Waka would give us their veggies from time to time to try, and we liked them all, but my favorite were the Japanese cucumbers; these have a unique flavor which we really love.

We started growing zinnias two years ago for customers to pick, because Sharon, one of our garden renters, grew some of the most beautiful zinnias we had ever seen. When she was finished with her garden, I gathered the seed from her zinnias and started a bed of my own, and now I grow hundreds for people to pick for table arrangements or gifts.

The U-Pick Garden lasts from the middle of June until the first or second week in August. The peak of our season is July 4th and two weeks after that.... most of the garden is in full production then and corn comes in around July 4th. Early (June) veggies are cabbage, broccoli, lettuce, spinach, kale, beets, carrots, herbs, and green beans (first crop). July 4th brings on tomatoes, corn, okra, eggplant, onions, and peppers.

Some plants need to be started in our greenhouse (e.g. tomatoes, peppers, and eggplant) because they need to be larger plants before you can put them in the ground, so they have a better chance of survival. Also our last day of frost is April 15th, so we try to have a good sturdy plant for transplanting, or we will not have these ready to pick by July 4th, our peak time.

We price our Garden plots as follows:

10x10 = $75
10x20 = $100
20x30 = $125 (best value)

Garden Rentals start in April and last until the first frost (roughly at the end of October).

One of the reasons we love what we do is because of the wonderful comments we hear about the experience as a whole. Our visitors learn a lot, because most of them have never gardened before. Although about 50% of our renters come back the next year, we do have turnover due to moving, starting raised beds in their own backyards (now that they know how to garden), and sadly… the death of a spouse. The Japanese family moved back to Japan…they were here on contract with Bridgestone for three years. A family moved to Canada for a new job…etc.

Another thing that really nurtures us is that people from all ethnic origins come to the U-Pick Garden and bring their entire family (from grandkids to great-grandparents). We are very welcoming and friendly to everyone and this kind of sets the tone for their visit. We invite the elderly folks to sit on our 12x60 back porch on our swings and rocking chairs, so they don't get overheated. It always reminds them of growing up as a child and they share stories about their past with the kids and grandkids. I think it's just as important to make new memories like picking at the farm too. We give all kids a freezer pop at the end (if its ok with their parents) as an extra treat to let them know we appreciate their visit. We provide milk crates to sit on in the green bean field, so it's easier than squatting for long periods of time. If it's REALLY HOT, we put canopies in the field to give some shade. Many of the people picking have conversations and meet each other for the first time.

One of my favorite memories is of Michelle and her two kids who came to the garden at 4:00 pm on a VERY HOT day. Michelle and the kids were dressed like they were going to a nice dinner that night, and were starting to pick on each other (as is typical for that time of day) and a little on the cranky side. The sun started to set past the outlying trees and the garden started to have shade. I talked to the kids about picking green beans, since they didn't know how…kind of like a treasure hunt. Since it was really hot, I got them a freezer pop while they continued to pick. A sprinkler was covering the squash plants nearby and her little boy started running under it and laughing. At first I thought Michelle was going to tell him to stop, but I explained that all the kids did that…so she let him. What a fun and relaxing afternoon that was for them and for me. Michelle and her kids come back every year…we have become good friends.

Twelve Herbs Every Gardener Should Have: (From Leigh)

When I was a young girl growing up on the farm in West Tennessee, I remember relatives who would tell me about picking something called poke salad. They would cook and season it as they would turnip greens, and eat it with beans and cornbread. I never really cared for poke salad, turnip greens or collard greens while I was growing up because I thought they tasted strong and I didn't really like the flavor. Today, I can't get enough of them, especially if they're seasoned with ham hock and splashed with a little pepper vinegar! I also remember talk of eating dandelions and other forage vegetables that we all had in our backyards. Even though I didn't want to try it as a kid, I was fascinated that people could eat food that grew just steps from their own back doors.

I guess this made sense if you think about it, though. When you live on a farm, it's not like you are exactly convenient to the local supermarket. It's a planned trip, with expenses of money and time just to get back and forth, not to mention facing food prices that are usually much higher than what you'd pay for food you grew yourself. Farmers tend to be self-reliant folks, who know the value of a dollar, and who all to often don't have that many dollars to throw around. Making the most of what Nature provided right off your doorstep was simply a practical solution to the questions of how to save time and stretch dollars.

When I came back to the farm in my 40's, I knew that I wanted to grow fresh herbs. Working for the Kroger Co. after college introduced me to fresh herbs, but I still didn't understand why they were important. The introduction of The Food Network has given many people a general understanding of how to use herbs in cooking, but most of the recipes still use the standards of basil, parsley, thyme, and chives. Don't get me wrong, there's nothing wrong with these. I knew I loved the flavor of fresh herbs but I wanted to know much more. I began to read the old Foxfire book series, which opened up a whole new world to me of learning how our ancestors used herbs in cooking, preserving and medicinally. (Olin's Uncle, Dennis Mitchell, first introduced me to the series and I was hooked: if you can get your hands on any of these books, they are definitely fascinating!)

Another, often overlooked, reason that herbs are an integral part of a healthy garden is because many of them attract beneficial insects ("Beneficial" because they act as predators and damaging parasites on insects that will otherwise ravage your garden and your produce). I'll be writing about beneficial insects another time, but just know for now (if you didn't already) that you cannot grow your food naturally (without pesticides/herbicides) unless you attract beneficial insects.

In 2010, Olin and I joined the Williamson County Master Gardeners Association (WCMGA) and we were introduced to Cindy Shapton, aka "The Cracked Pot Gardener". Cindy is herself a certified Master Gardener, herbalist, consultant and garden designer for commercial and residential clients, a writer and speaker. She was a past president of the WCMGA and a regular speaker, but more than that she was the most knowledgeable person I had ever met concerning growing and using herbs both for culinary and medicinal purposes. I was and remain fascinated by the sheer amount of knowledge she had on the history of herbs and their uses.

Cindy had written a book in 2007, called *The Cracked Pot Herb Book: Simple Ways to Incorporate Herbs into Everyday Life*, which has been very well received by anyone lucky enough to procure a copy. I still use Cindy's book regularly for both the recipes and the background information and history she shares about herbs.

In 2011, when we opened Stoney Creek Farm to the public, Cindy Shapton was one of the first speakers we engaged to give a seminar specifically on herbs. She is a delightful speaker and uses humor to deliver all of her valuable information. Below are some nuggets that she has shared in her classes at our farm:

The Romans used coriander (the seed of cilantro) as a spice and meat preservative. They in turn adopted this practice from Eastern traders, especially those from faraway India, who had been using this herb as a preservative and medicine for centuries.

Dill also goes back in history to biblical times, where it was used as a medicine to remedy colic, flatulence, estrogen deficiency, digestive problems, and bad breath.

If you've never tried a small leaf of sage on a Ritz cracker with cream cheese, you are missing out! It makes the greatest appetizer.

Oregano leaves makes a great tea that can soothe your throat during cold season.

Many plants that we think of as weeds are actually herbs. For instance, Chickweed is loaded with vitamins A, B, and C, calcium, phosphorus, potassium, and zinc. The Dandelions you may try to kill off on your lawns are a diuretic, great for weight loss and high blood pressure, and contain mega amounts of vitamins and minerals. They may also be beneficial in cancer prevention and therapy: Who knew?

Lemon Balm contains citronella in the leaves and works as an insect repellent when you rub it on your skin. Cindy also has a wonderful lemon balm bread recipe in her book.

These are the twelve basic herbs that I believe everyone should have in their garden and these are the ones that I grow for the public and myself:

1. Basil - this is my favorite just because it's so darned tasty and you can use it in almost anything, especially fresh pesto. I also love basil because it's a companion plant for my tomatoes. It helps deter evil insects with its smell.

2. Oregano - I use it in all my Italian recipes, but just a little goes a long way. I also use it in the winter during cold season, to brew in a tea and drink hot... helps sore throats.

3. Rosemary - in our growing area only the ARP variety will sustain through the winter. Rosemary potatoes, Rosemary chicken, and sprinkling Rosemary in salad all yield very tasty recipes.

4. Lemon Balm - be sure to grow lemon balm with a barrier around it because it is invasive and left to itself will take over your entire garden. But I love lemon balm to flavor water or tea, in homemade bread, and to use as an insect repellent on my skin during the summer. (Mosquitoes love me.)

5. Cilantro - I am a salsa nut and you can't make fresh salsa without it. It hates hot weather in the summer, but just know that it will reseed itself in the fall for fresher salsa.

6. Dill - great in salads and homemade pickles, but best of all, a host plant for butterflies.

7. Mint - any variety is great (but also very invasive) and can be used in fruit salads, jellies, and numerous drink recipes.

8. Parsley - "the herb of champions" it compliments other herbs by helping balance out strongly flavored ones.

9. Nasturtium - beautiful flowers and spicy leaves that can be eaten in salads.

10. Sage - I love the flavor all year round...in appetizers, on meat dishes, stuffing and more.

11. Garlic - I know, I know, it's not an herb, but I grow it in my herb garden, so I think everyone should have it. I use it sparingly in most dishes for flavor. I've also read that it kills bacteria, lowers cholesterol, and is a natural antibiotic.

12. Comfrey - mostly medicinal, use externally on the skin as a natural Band-Aid. Also, comfrey leaves in a bucket with water (compost tea) makes a wonderful liquid fertilizer after it sits a few days.

Bonus Note: One herb that is particularly helpful for people with migraines is **Feverfew**. I grew it one year, but I do not have migraines, so I gave it to someone who did.

It's important to know that to keep many of your herbs growing throughout the summer, you will need to trim the flowers from the herbs on a regular basis. This practice is especially important on basil and cilantro. The flowers are the plant's way of starting to regenerate itself for the next season by making seed. Keeping the flowers trimmed will prolong the life of the herb.

Preserving Herbs for the Winter:

I don't preserve nasturtium or comfrey, but I dry most of my herbs in a dehydrator or tie I them in bundles and hang them in the garage during the winter months. If you do this, just make sure your garage is cool and dry, not moist, because the herbs will mold in a moist environment. Two herbs that I freeze are Mint and Basil, because I think they taste better frozen than dried. I simply pick the leaves off the stems, wash them thoroughly, pat them dry with paper towels and put them in plastic freezer bags to store in the freezer. To use them, just take out a small frozen amount and crush into your recipe. The leaves will be crunchy, so it makes it easy to crush them.

By now you probably realize that there is much more I could say about herbs than I have room for here, but I definitely enjoy growing them, and get a lot of use out of them. If you aren't yet growing herbs in your garden, I'd strongly recommend you start. We offer cuttings at our farm that can help you do this. If you'd like to know what a real expert has to say about herbs, I would strongly recommend that you visit Cindy Shapton's website, www.crackedpotgardener.com to get an astounding amount of information on her beloved herbs, as well as homesteading and organic practices. (You can also purchase Cindy's book on her website.)

You can use almost any container to grow herbs, and are limited only by your imagination: wheelbarrows, old sinks, etc. Deep containers only need about 6-8 inches of soil, so use your recyclables, such as two-liter bottles, milk jugs, etc. (non-decomposable) or decomposable items such as old pots (cardboard kind).

Watering Your Plants:

For in-ground gardens, 1 inch of water per week is required. Rainwater is always preferred, but sometimes Mother Nature doesn't cooperate. We keep a rain gauge to be able to measure rain each week and communicate with our garden renters on the amount of rainfall.

For raised beds, the rainfall required is similar, but may require a little more, due to the soil drying out faster. If you use a soil mixture of half compost and half topsoil, your plants will need 1 ½ to 2 inches of water per week (you can approximate about one quart a plant for one inch a week). If your raised bed is using the Square Foot Garden Mix (Mel's Mix), then he says you cannot overwater it. That must be because of all the drainage materials in this mix.

Regardless of what type of garden you have… don't water each day, usually every 3 days is fine and if it's very hot and dry, otherwise once a week is ok. Overwatering can ruin plants, as it gives them "wet feet" and their roots don't progress. Rainwater is the best source of water, due to lack of chlorine.

Protecting Your Plants Without Pesticides:

When we started, Leigh's Uncle told her she needed to have a chemical license if she was going to start a farm, in case she needed stronger pesticides than what they carried in the stores. Who would have known that this certification would cause a USDA farm inspection? AND we never used the stronger chemicals! USDA does not usually test small farms (and we are happy to say that we passed this inspection twice). Fortunately, after the chemical license expired, the farm stopped being inspected.

Bottom line: as with so many other regulatory bodies, if you have chemical licenses, the USDA may come and see if you are using toxic chemicals.

Insects can cause a wide variety of plant diseases, and the Ag. Extension in your state can provide you with a long list of plant pests, and pest removal strategies, including pesticides. Instead of pesticides we use flowers to attract beneficial insects, as one of the best ways to reduce insect pests is to introduce other insects into your garden that will prey upon the pests you have, while leaving your plants alone.

Although this sounds great in theory, you need to be careful how you do this, as you can't just put insects in the garden, they will fly away. SO you need to develop a strategy to attract them. Don't buy the ladybeetles you'll find advertised online. You will be buying convergent beetles. They don't know to stay in your yard: they are predators! They'll fly away unless you learn to attract them properly.

True insects have three pairs of legs (spiders are not insects). Fly larvae are called maggots, and look like grubs, not flies.

Insects don't really have brains, they have a ganglion, so they can't feel emotions as we know them. We humans tend to project our human emotions onto them. You've heard the expression: "angry as a hornets nest." While the hornets seem "angry" to us, this is actually an emotion that is far too complex for them to feel. The "angry hornet" swarm is essentially a series of hormonal and other chemical responses to environmental threat stimuli. Which doesn't make it hurt any less when they sting you, just don't take it personally.

Insects see in a different light spectrum than we do, and can see UV light, which is invisible to us. We say that their vision is "blue-shifted." So a flower that looks white to us looks blue to an insect, and one which looks red to us will look black, because as they can see more into the blue range they lose the ability to see in the red range.

There are an incredible number of insects, and insect species, in the world. In North America, for example, we have over 450 species of lady beetle, and some don't even look like the classic red/orange color with black spots.

Insects don't live a very long time, especially in the adult form, which typically only exists to reproduce more eggs, which turn into larvae, etc. Mayflies only live a day (Order Ephemeroptera: life is truly ephemeral for them).

The longest-lived insects in North America are the 13 year and 17 year cicadas. The larval stage is what lives for 13 or 17 years, developing oh so slowly in the ground. The adults live only a month or so.

The lady beetles we discussed above are all predators with chewing mouthparts. They don't eat plants, but need to eat other insects. So we need to entice the female insects in to feed so they will lay their eggs in strategic spots, which become the larvae you need to control the pests. Sometimes there will be no pests and the insects move on.

The Flower/Insect Dance:

Now, many of the insects we'd like to attract have little tiny mouthparts, so they need flowers where the nectar is readily available, as they can't access the deep, tubular type flowers.

Those latter flowers are designed more for honeybees bumble bees, etc. which have longer tongues. The insects we want need readily available nectar. You also need a variety of flowers, in order to attract a variety of beneficial insects, including deep tubular flowers for bumble bees, honey bees, etc. as well as the flowers where the nectar is closer to the surface for the parasitic wasps, for example.

Flowers actually have little lines in the UV spectrum (which we can't see) pointing the bee to the nectar source, like an airport runway at night. So insects and flowers have evolved together so there is a real association between them. That's why if certain species of insects disappear we will lose certain species of plants, and if we lose certain species of plants we will lose the insects that feed on them.

Nectar is the food made via photosynthesis mixed with nutrients and water taken up from the soil through the roots. Nectar is basically plant sap, and is exuded out near the flowers because that's where the insects go. It's the "reward" because some plants need their pollen to be moved to another flower. Some plants are not self-fertile (cannot pollinate themselves) need pollen from another plant of the same species, which insects provide by flitting from flower to flower.

Nectar is the payoff for the insect to make this effort. Insects literally get food in return for facilitating plant sex!

The female part of the flower is the ovary. Stigma, style, and pistil are the other female parts of the flower). The stamen and anther, etc. comprise the male parts. Some vegetables (squash for instance) have male and female flowers, so the female flowers do not have any of the male parts, and vice versa. Pollen is microscopic powder on top of the anther, and is necessary for the fertilization of the female flower. Male flowers appear first with squash, so people will get all excited when they see a ton of flowers because they think they are going to get a lot of squash. Wrong! They have a lot of male flowers. Female flowers appear later. Bees go looking for pollen: they can't tell between male and female flowers, so they brush up against the pollen. When they don't find nectar, the bee will move to a female flower, find nectar, and mechanically transfer the pollen to the female flower, and fertilizes it.

If you see a cucumber or squash that doesn't do very well, maybe looks deformed, that may well be due to incomplete fertilization. Mission of all plants is to make seed. Plant will not expend energy on stuff that won't produce seed. That's why we "deadhead" dead flowers on certain plants, to encourage more flowering and thereby more fruit production.

Leaves, sepals (immature petals), form the flower petals. All the petals together in the flower are called the corona.

So which insects will help us to reduce other insect pests, and what flowers do they like to feed on?

Beneficial Insects:

Larval Lady Beetles: Most insects, once they hatch from an egg, are in a stage known as a larva. This then goes through a stage where it will eventually turn into a completely different insect, a life cycle known as complete metamorphosis. Larva can look completely different from adults.

Green Lacewing: (smaller one is brown lacewing). Lacewings are excellent protection for a lot of plants. It will look like they are eating your plants, but aren't. The adults, who only live a few weeks, have chewing mouthparts, but the female is the one that needs nectar. They lay eggs on a little stalk, on the bottom of a leaf, which hides them from predators.

The larval stage has fangs. They'll grasp the prey insect, and inject digestive juices into their prey. Digestion occurs outside the body, and then they suck the juices out. Lacewing larvae are excellent predators for aphids. In fact we buy lacewing eggs to place on our tomato plants to eradicate aphid infestations.

Hover Fly: This insect has its name because it hovers over flowers, it resembles a bee, but bees need to be in motion, they don't hover. Sometimes they get tired and may alight on your finger. They don't have mouthparts or stings. They are very tiny. Adult lives a year or less.

The hover fly will look for small colony of aphids and lay an egg.

The eggs will hatch into blind, legless larvae, which then begin to crawl, so the eggs need to be laid close to food source. Aphids will stay on leaf, or wherever, unaware of the hover fly larvae predation going on around them. The adult female is not eating the aphids; it is the larva that does this.

Flies: are also important because they clean up the mess when an animal dies. You can think of flies as the buzzards of the insect class.

Tachinid Wasps:

Parasatoid wasps are smaller than a gnat; insert their eggs into the body of an aphid without killing it. The female does not feed on other insects; she needs nectar. The egg receives its protein from the "infected" host insect. Will consume from the inside of the body and eventually kill it (which is what you want).

They have a spongy mouthpart to suck up nectar. The female lays her egg not on the plant, but lays sticky eggs right onto the host insect (uses the oopositor, literally egg depositor). Just like the movie alien, the eggs hatch, and the larva invades the body of the host insect and starts feeding, but not too much too quickly, as they don't want to kill it right away.

When the larva is ready, it can pupate in some form of cocoon (dormant) but not all insects pupate. A parasite will not kill its host. So, consider you may have moth eggs, and you know the moth will turn into a caterpillar, which may eat your vegetables. So this little tiny wasp will lay her egg inside the moth egg (remember this is very small).

All of this is part of the energy cycle: Light> Plant> Herbivore> Carnivore. Light becomes, plant, becomes animal, animal becomes prey, and so on.

The parasitic wasp adult emerges from the calcified exoskeleton of now-dead host, and begins feeding on nectar to fuel the source for other insect host sites where it can lay its eggs.

Almost every plant outside has a different species of aphid that will attack it. So some wasps are very host specific and only attack certain aphids.

Remember: If you spray the aphids, you will kill the wasps too.

Wasps can insert 50 or more eggs onto a caterpillar. To the wasp, the caterpillar is huge!

Wasp larvae can just poke their way out of the caterpillar. Caterpillar will stop feeding within a couple of days and die, especially due to the trauma from the larva leaving its body. Larva will spin a silk cocoon on the caterpillar's outside, and pupate there. The larva inside the cocoon actually breaks down into a liquid and reforms into the adult.

Other Insect Predators We Like:

When you are outside and suddenly feel a little sting on the back of your hand, its probably a little tiny true bug, all bugs have beaks so you feel their bites no matter how small it is.

Damsel Bugs are also good insect predators.

Stink Bugs, aka spine soldier bugs, are predaceous, and will attack caterpillars.

The **Tiger Beetle** will run and jump on prey even though it can fly. They like really sunny spots. They aren't attracted to flowers themselves but hang around flowers because their prey often is attracted to the flowers.

Beneficial Flowers:

The best flowering plant ever for attracting beneficial insects is called buckwheat. You can buy the seed at a farm store like a co-op. It is not usually available in little bags; they will have it in massive amounts. Go into your local co-op farm store and ask for buckwheat seed. They should go in the back, and pour it out into a little brown lunch bag, weigh it, etc. If your local co-op only sells the large 50 lb. bags of seed, then order it online from a seed company. Buckwheat is a nice flowering plant, with nectar ready available.

Trivia fact: Buckwheat pancakes are made from buckwheat flour, not wheat flour.

Buckwheat is best placed an inch in the ground near your plant. Needs to be on the center and edges of your garden. Bugs attack garden edges first, so your beneficial-attractive plants should be on the edges as well.

Buckwheat is an annual that should be planted when weather warms up (around first of May). It has a triangular seed. This plant, while accessible to smaller insects, is also a magnet for honeybees, due to its high quality nectar. Does a very nice job of controlling insect pests on tomato plants (white flies, aphids, thrips, etc.). Plant three or four buckwheat seeds next to the tomato plant. Buckwheat can germinate in about 3-4 days, in 2-3 weeks it will start flowering, and draw in beneficial insects. Don't over-sow the buckwheat or it may make the tomato plant too moist.

In a grape orchard, you should plant buckwheat in between the grape vines. The pest pressure will drop off as you build up your beneficial insect population. One guy who owned a greenhouse was having a lot of problems with white flies. He introduced buckwheat into the greenhouse and completely got rid of them. In an enclosed environment you can often see 100% control (because the beneficial insects do not escape).

Sweet Alyssa, often used as an ornamental, comes in very light blues, and pinkish hues as well. It is another very useful plant for attracting beneficial insects. It has a very shallow flower, so its nectar is accessible, which really attracts hover flies, with their sponge-type mouthparts, and parasitic wasps. Grows well on the edge of a garden that gets full sun. Will reseed.

Bachelor's Button (aka Corn Flower): Even before it flowers, this plant has extra-nectary floral glands. This means that even before it flowers, insects will visit this plant. It is easy to collect seed from it, and it will also re-seed. Cornflowers can be planted alone or with poppies. Poppy seeds have to be put down in fall (cold stratification). Daisies are also good for attracting beneficials.

Trivia Fact: As an FYI, six hours is considered "full sun" light for flowers. Fruit (including tomatoes) need more sun.

Cosmos is also easy to grow, pretty, will re-seed, drought and heat tolerant, a plant that thrives on neglect, good for beneficials.

Plains Coreopsis and **Moonbeam Coreopsis** will bloom, and bloom, and bloom, do pretty well with neglect, and attract beneficials.

Cat mint (not nip): This is a very drought tolerant plant, which grows 3 feet tall and wide. It is a perennial type of shrub that butterflies and bees really like. Don't do anything to it until it's through blooming, just shear it back, and it will re-bloom.

When you get into late season, it's very critical that honeybees and bumblebees have a good food source to survive the winter. **Goldenrod** blooms at the same time as ragweed, and is the same color, but does not cause hay fever. Its pollen is not airborne. Goldenrod is a late season bloomer (late summer into fall).

Honeybees don't preferably visit corn; the nectar is too low nutrient for them. Some of the plants that have been crossbred to produce big flowers with vibrant colors sometimes come at the price of low-nutrient nectar. So bees don't thrive as well with these "overbred" plants. Low nutrient nectar means smaller colonies and lower survival rates over the winter.

Perennial Sunflowers, which are actually shrubs that can grow tall, should be planted by themselves. They bloom in October. Plant zebra grass around it to help support it.

You can also try throwing wildflower seeds around the edge of your garden to attract beneficials. You can get early blooming, cold resistant wildflowers all the way through others that will bloom into the fall, so you can get a whole series of wildflower blooms all the way through the year. Once you get them established, you can just leave them alone.

We have found that planting beneficial flowers, to attract beneficial insects, is an effective tactic for minimizing garden pests without the use of pesticides. As well as being consistent with the sustainable farming philosophy it has the additional advantage of supplementing the beauty and overall health of your garden.

6. THE BUZZ ABOUT BEES

We believe we need to leave the earth better than we found it. One way to do that is to save our bees. Pollination is so important for our planet and bees are disappearing from the earth at a rapid pace due to many factors. It is common knowledge that at least 1/3 of every bite of food you eat is due to the work of bees and other pollinators. Did you know that bees are the only insects that produce a food that humans eat? Honey is the only food that includes everything to sustain life (enzymes, vitamins, minerals, and water). It also contains 'pinocembrin' which is an antioxidant that improves brain functioning. I hope this chapter will encourage you to get involved in saving our bees from extinction.

Honey Bees

As we began our Dirt Rich journey, we realized how important pollination is for both the U-Pick Garden and Garden Rental Plots. We had a neighbor about ½ mile down the road who had multiple bee hives and sold local honey. These bees visited our farm daily during the spring and summer months and fully pollinated all of our vegetables and fruits…what a great relationship…free pollination! We had lots of other pollinators, but the bees, as we found out, were the top contributors.

About 4 years after we opened Stoney Creek Farm to the public, the County Maintenance Crew sprayed pesticides on the county road "right of way" too close to our neighbor's bees and wiped out all of his hives, as well as his local honey business. We started to notice a reduction in production of our vegetables and fruit due to losing the honey bees, so we began our research on beekeeping.

Since we already had full schedules, beekeeping was not something we could add easily and we wanted to make sure bees would be cared for in a responsible manner. We researched several options:

1. Rent bee hives from a responsible beekeeper – this proved to be fairly expensive at $100 per month and was not a viable option for us.
2. Work with a local honey supplier to provide bees and sell their honey – we were able to sell the local honey, but unable to get the supplier to locate bees on our farm.
3. Find a volunteer who was interested in bee keeping at our farm – this option was viable. We bought all supplies including bees, hives, suits, and accessories and our volunteer agreed to care for the bees. Although this option was the most expensive up-front cost of the three, we felt this one was the most sustainable and cost effective in the long run.

Then we met Cathi Clarke, who was a Godsend for us. Cathi's son, Grant, who had a garden plot rental at the farm, introduced her to us and our relationship began. Cathi lived in an apartment and was the primary caretaker for her adult mentally challenged daughter. At first Cathi just wanted to volunteer and be able to bring her adult daughter to the farm for some fresh air and sunshine. Then we found out that she had always wanted to have honey bees and learn how to care for them…hard to do in an apartment setting. Some people would say that's a coincidence, but I know better…Cathi was sent to us.

Cathi agreed to be our beekeeper volunteer and we began our beekeeping adventure. Cathi insisted on paying for her training class, and we paid for everything else. Her job would be to take care of the bees and our job was to provide her with everything she needed to do so.

Beekeeping 101

Cathi attended a recommended, all-natural beekeeping class one weekend in February to learn about the care and handling of the bees. Cathi's weekend class cost $99 but classes can cost up to $300 depending on the area.

The major points Cathi learned during the weekend of training are listed below:

- Which Hives and Tools are recommended in the care and handling of honey bees
- The two different methods to buy a starter hive: **1) Nucleus Colony**: Includes queen, and several thousand bees on frames which you can simply transfer to your hive. **2) Packaged Bees**: Includes worker bees shipped in a screened box with 2 to 4 pounds of worker bees and the queen suspended in a separate cage. After the syrup is removed, the bees are shaken into an empty hive and the queen cage is suspended between frames. Eventually the worker bees accept the queen and eat through the ends of the queen cage to release her.
- How to locate the ideal Apiary or Bee Yard in the proper location with the essential elements such as food and water source, sun/shade, wind protection, air circulation and more
- Beekeeping regulations and registration for your hives
- Feeding and supplementation of the Hives to keep them healthy
- Different Races or Breeds of Bees such as Italian, Buckfast, Russian and more
- Various Methods of Pest control with Varroa Mites, Hive Beetles and Wax Moths
- Goals for Honey Production with 100 pounds or more of surplus honey being the most desirable and 50 - 60 pounds the norm. These goals are for the future, not for beginning beekeepers.
- Types of Beekeeping Protective Gear such as hats, helmets, gloves, clothing and boots

- How to inspect the hives, and find the queen and elements necessary for her care.

It was a whirlwind weekend with an overwhelming amount of information for Cathi to absorb. She was apprehensive, but excited about being able accomplish one of the 'bucket list' goals for her life. So along with Cathi, we began our beekeeping adventure.

At the weekend beekeeping retreat, Cathi purchased the following items to begin the Stoney Creek Farm Apiary:

- **Two Langstroth Hive Kits** (One kit consists of 4 Medium Supers, 1 Feeder Station, and an Outer Cover): $426
- **One Beginner Tool Kit** (Brush, Smoker, Hive Tool, Leather Gloves, Frame Grip, 3 Beetle Blasters): $100
- **Frame Holder:** $18
- **Ventilated Jacket with Veil:** $82.50
    (Note: The full ventilated body suit cost $125)
- **Two Nucleus Hives**: $320

Total Cost for Two Hives: $928.50

Olin also built an elevated deck and shelter for the hives, so they would be protected from storms and flooding water which cost about $60. At almost $1,000 for two hives, which is the cost we expected, this option was still overall the least expensive option and the most sustainable one.

After the bees were delivered in May, we registered the hives with the state of Tennessee. Registration for bee hives is required, so that serious bee diseases and colony collapse can be documented for records and statistics. Cathi visited the hives at least 3 times a week to make sure everything was going well. The bottom super (or brooder box) held the nucleus colony. She inspected the hives by taking out frames and searching for the queen every couple of weeks at first and was careful not to mash the queen during this process. Killing the queen is one of the number one issues with new beekeepers.

During the summer months, the hives had a tremendous war going on with predatory insects. Hive Beetles, wasps, yellow jackets, ants, carpenter bees and later, Varroa Mites created a tough environment for the new hives. These predatory insects attack the hives in multiple ways: robbing honey, eating or carrying off new bee larvae, weakening new bees with virus and bacteria transmission, and laying predatory eggs in brooder cells. Cathi fought the predators with natural treatments such as oxalic acid, diatomaceous earth (DE), and even Crisco, but the hive beetles would not give up. Finally, after many weeks of trying to eradicate the beetles, she used a recommended encased pesticide that would not hurt the bees, but attracted and eliminated the beetles. Fortunately, she was able to remove the beetle issue without harm to the bees or honey.

As the brooder super started filling up with more new bees and honey, she would add another medium super with frames to the top of the brooder box after it was about 70-80% full. To be clear, 'supers' are the boxes with frames that hold the bees and honey. One hive appeared to be producing at a faster rate than the other, so she added the medium supers at different times to each hive. After the hives had grown to 4 supers, in September, it appeared that they were finished for the summer season and Cathi began to get them ready for winter. The recommendation by class teachers was to take no honey from the hive in the first year, so that the bees had plenty of food for the winter and the ability to thrive into the New Year.

In September, Cathi was inspecting the hives and discovered that both queens had left the hives. She did not find any larvae queen cells, which appear like 'peanuts'; queen eggs are larger than worker bee cells. We immediately ordered new queens for the hives at $60 each, but alas, they both died within 2 weeks. Both queens were put in the hives with cages, so that the bees could accept them into the hive, but we feel that they were weak queens and that characteristic is probably the reason they did not survive. Honey bees can be weakened by many things: genetics, bacteria or viral disease, predators, and in this case, it could have been any or all of these.

About this same time, Cathi noticed a Varroa Mite infestation in the hives. She began treating the hives for the pests, but to no avail.

Within a few weeks, the majority of bees left the hives and we suffered a condition called 'colony collapse'. To explain how the Varroa Mites attack honey bees, they attach themselves to the bee larvae and pass disease (bacteria or viral) that weakens their immune system. These mites originated in Asia, established in Africa and Europe to eventually spread around the world. The U.S. detected the mites on honey bees in 1987 and beekeepers have been struggling to eradicate them since then.

Needless to say, we were crushed…all that work…all that expense! But most of all, we were disappointed because our honey bees were gone! Little did we know that the State of Tennessee lost 78% of all beehives in 2017. We were not alone! Most of these beehives were lost to well established beekeepers with numerous hives and booming businesses. Farm Bureau reported on the loss of hives and interviewed Barry Richards, the President of the Tennessee Beekeepers Association, who mentioned the infestation of Varroa Mites as well as unintentional pesticide drift from agricultural crops. If you would like to learn more about this phenomenon, this Farm Bureau article "A Dwindling Buzz" is very enlightening: https://www.tnfarmbureau.org/a-dwindling-buzz.

It was a great learning experience and we will never regret putting in the hives. We wanted to continue beekeeping and allow Cathi to expand her knowledge and opportunities with honeybees. We had even discussed producing pollen, lip balm and other beeswax products for sale. Also, Cathi was able to teach an 'Introduction to Beekeeping' Class for the community about the costs and work involved in hosting an Apiary. The class was very well received and we had hoped to continue more learning opportunities for the public. Cathi cleaned and stored the hives in our shop area to keep wax moths from infiltrating the hives and eating the frame wax.

At the end of the year, Cathi had to relocate to East Tennessee and we are still searching for either another volunteer beekeeper or other pollination options. We still keep in touch with Cathi and hope someday, she will be able to return to the area. Olin and I also joined the Middle Tennessee Beekeeper's Association last year to keep updated on beehive activity across the state. We have made some terrific contacts that may give us other pollination opportunities.

One of our highly recommended publications is the University of Tennessee's 'Beekeeping in Tennessee', which could be used in most states for reference.

The free publication is found at the UT publication site: https://extension.tennessee.edu/publications/Pages/default.aspx

Simply enter PB1745 in the search bar to download the publication.

Although beekeeping is not for everyone, it is definitely worth investigating. Visiting your local beekeeping association and finding out more about how to save our honeybees is a valuable learning activity for every age group and walk of life.

Solitary Bees

Two years before we bought our honeybees, Jay Williams, Director of Farm Operations, Crown Bees approached us about being a test program for Solitary Bees (Mason and Leafcutter Bees) at our farm. We paid a small amount of money to cover his expenses, and Jay put two hive boxes of Leaf Cutter Bees on our property to hopefully increase our pollination rates. After the season was over, I wrote the following blog article on our website:

Leaf Cutter Bees – Superhero Pollinators!

When Jay Williams from Williams Honey Farm approached us about a pollination test this Summer season for Solitary Bees (Mason & Leaf Cutter Bees), we didn't really know what to expect, but he made it very easy. Jay basically did all the work and we reaped all the benefits. We only paid him for cost of the bees and materials. He placed two T-Post Hives on our farm. One T-post Hive was in the area of our U-Pick Community Garden and the other post hive was in our rental gardens. (We rent plots to local people who are either learning how to garden or do not have the space at their homes or apartment communities.) Jay placed approximately 1,000 Leaf Cutter cocoons and bees at each T-Post Hive for the test.

He placed the box and cocoons in early June and they began their pollination cycle. We have never seen anything like it before! We are only estimating, but feel that they at least tripled our pollination rate. We began to feel overwhelmed because we do not have a large enough staff (just the two of us and two volunteers) to keep up with the production of vegetables we were picking every day...much more than in the previous 5 years we have been open. We started out with 6 rows of green beans (4 rows less than last year) and we were not able to pick all of the green beans on two of the rows, before they got dry on the vine...there were just so many beans. We are determined next year to be more prepared, because we lost a lot of veggies...we just couldn't harvest it all!

We sold more squash, zucchini, tomatoes, broccoli, Brussel sprouts, cabbage, and berries than any previous year we have been open and we feel it is due in a large part to the increased pollination of the leaf cutter bees.

We opened the garden in mid-June and closed in 6 weeks, 2 weeks earlier than usual. Increased pollination may have played a part, but the heat and excessive rain definitely accelerated plant deterioration.

Even though we closed two weeks earlier than usual...we still increased our sales 35% above 2015 *(and 2015 was higher than any previous year). We had more produce than we could sell so, we also donated almost 1,000 pounds of produce (estimated worth of $1,000) to OneGenAway (www.onegenaway.com) which distributes food throughout our community to the needy and homeless. We felt very blessed this year!.*

If you have an interest in getting some Solitary Bees (Mason and/or Leaf Cutter) for your farm, garden or landscape, we definitely recommend Jay Williams and his little Super Hero Pollinators. Contact him at jay@crownbees.com.

As you can read from the blog, we were VERY HAPPY with the results of our pollination test. We continue to use Leaf Cutter bees to pollinate our crops and now have a sustainable program with Crown Bees. The sustainable program involves paying for a crate/house, 6 boxes with pencil size holes for egg laying, a cocoon releaser and chicken wire cover (to prevent bird predation). The first year we received three distributions of leafcutter cocoons two weeks apart through the mail. Leaf Cutters have a specific lifecycle that involves cutting a tiny piece of leaf and then using it to encapsulate their larvae in a cocoon inside the pencil-size holes of the boxes.

The Leaf Cutter Life Cycle:

- Adults emerge from "leaf cocoons"
- Mating occurs
- Feeding and Pollination
- Lay eggs inside leaf cocoons

After their Summer life cycle is over, we collect the boxes and place them in screen bags (to prevent moths from infesting the boxes, and laying eggs which eventually hatch into caterpillars that eat the leafcutter larvae). The boxes are kept in a cool, dry environment over the winter and the cocoons are harvested from the boxes in April. We put out the cocoons in early June, when produce and berries are blooming and need pollination. The bees only travel about 300 – 400 feet, so it's important to locate your bee crate/home in a convenient location to the produce and fruit. We feel strongly that we at least triple our pollination rate by using leafcutters and the cost is very minimal.

Besides the tremendous increase in pollination, other reasons we love leafcutter bees are: they don't sting, they are sustainable, they are native to our area, and they have a mutually symbiotic relationship with honeybees (they both benefit from the relationship).

On our Facebook Page, we have a leafcutter video to show active leafcutter bees with the crate/house and egg laying boxes: https://www.facebook.com/stoneycreekfarmtennessee/videos/9327 51576879580/

If you want to learn more about Solitary Bees and how your landscape or garden can benefit from using them, check out the Crown Bee website: www.crownbees.com.

Plants that Attract Bees

If you want to attract bees to your garden or property, plant native bushes and flowers that feed the bees. These are also known as Bee Forage Plants. Below is a list of plants (not all-inclusive) that work in numerous gardening zones, but it is important to check your zone to make sure they are hardy for your area.

Annuals
Arugula
Basil
Borage
Buckwheat
Canola (Rapeseed)
Cleome
Cornflower
Flax
Cosmos
Crimson Clover
Holy Basil
Mustard
Sunflower
Poppies
Verbena
Zinnia

Perennials

Spring Bulbs
Anise Hyssop
Asters
Berries
Catmint
Chives
Comfrey
Coreopsis
Dandelion
Echinacea
Gaillardia
Globe Thistle
Goldenrod
Hazelnut
Hyssop

Lavender
Melissa
Mint
Monardo
Motherwort
Obedient Plant
Oregano
Plantain
Pussy Willow
Rose Mallow
Rosemary
Sage
Sedum
Sunflower (perennial)
Sweet Clover
Thyme
Wild Rose
White Clover
Verbena (perennial)

Trees

Tulip Poplar
Linden
Black Locust
Sourwood
Fruit Trees

Although this is not an all-inclusive list of bee forage plants, it will give you an idea of the many options available for planting in your garden or landscape. Once these plants, bushes and trees are established in your area, they will provide generous amounts of pollen and nectar for your native bee population.

7. ANIMALS FOR FUN, FOOD, AND PROFIT

Disclaimer: *We are not experts in the farm animal field. We are providing some general information on farm animals, but you should always check with your local veterinarian prior to administration of any medical treatment (topical or oral) for your farm animals.*

What would a farm be without its animals? Even though we have a plant-based operation as the draw to our farm, we do raise chickens (and will try to reintroduce more goats, eventually, as well).

But your passion may require you to raise certain type of animals on your farm, and if we didn't supply with at least some information to help guide you in those decisions, this book would fall short of its goal of helping you match your farming activity with your passion.

So here are some of the animals that we know a little about. Our daughter, Dr. Allison Mallard, a graduate of the UT College of Veterinary Medicine, helped tremendously with putting together the majority of this information. Again, it's by no means an exhaustive list, but hopefully enough information to begin with:

Dogs:

When having dogs on a farm, it's important to know whether you want them as working dogs or pets. Try not to mix these roles, as they will get confused. Consider taking a training class on how to train a dog, and go through it with yours. You need to be the alpha, and have the bond with you.

Farm-Friendly Dog Breeds:

1) Great Pyrenees: These "nannying dogs" are raised as herding and guarding dogs, and will guard livestock from pretty much anything (wolves to people). They may be pretty shy, possibly even with owners, so it's best to ensure they know they are working dogs and not pets. Pyrenees are big and woolly, but do not shed very much. They can adjust to almost any temperature and climate. Pyrenees are good with all livestock, and love other animals (except for threats). These dogs are easy to take care of, and are a very popular breed for farm work.

2) Border Collie: This breed is more like a herding and gathering (vs. guarding) dog. They are very intelligent and energetic, so they need to be worked, otherwise they can get into mischief: they need to be kept challenged. Border collies are very loyal, and love to please.

3) German Shepherd: You may think of these dogs mostly as K9/FBI dogs, but they were first raised as shepherd's dogs (hence the name). Shepherds are very good at guarding, They are not really the herding type, but are very good at keeping everyone safe on the farm. They are very loyal, and though often sweet-tempered, they can be territorial and very protective, so you'll need to train them young on how to act with strangers.

4) Corgi: Don't let their small size fool you! Corgis were bred to snap at cattle heels and herd them, and so are not at all afraid of larger animals. Because of the general domestication of the breed, which now has even shorter legs, they are probably better for small ruminants and perhaps chickens. Corgis are very smart as well.

5) Rottweiler: Not many people know that these dogs have been bred as guarding, territorial animals since Roman times. They are great nannying dogs, like Great P's, but are very territorial and they need to be introduced to strangers slowly. You need to be there, otherwise they may, if not attack, shall we say display their territorial nature. So Rottweilers, while great at what they do, and potentially very gentle and loving, because of the "Cujo" mystique make many people hesitant to use them.

6) Australian Cattle Dog: This is another really smart herding breed, and not so much a guarding breed to scare predators away. They will keep livestock together and on the property. These dogs are very fast and nimble, and typically weigh only about 30-40 lbs. max. They are very fast and smart, and are another breed that you need to keep engaged. In fact, many of these breeds that can be used with effect on the farm do not do so well in urban settings/apartments, etc., and will tear stuff up because it is difficult to keep them active enough and their minds engaged enough. You really need to "wear them out."

7) English Sheep Dogs: These dogs are bred to care for sheep, and are one of the oldest and well-known herding dogs. They are also one of the most successful farm helpers, due to their strength and agility. They will stand up to almost any predator, but also have a very sweet temperament and are very loving. They have a thick coat, but this is breathable, so they don't get super-hot and can do well in hot summers. Contrary to what you might think, they do not require a whole lot of coat management. They will get shaggy if they are outdoors a lot, but a trim at a vet's office once or twice a year should be enough to deal with this, and won't cost you much.

8) Bernese Mountain Dog: These are very similar to the Great Pyrenees, and are bred mainly for guarding. They are very attentive to what they do, but perhaps not as agile as some other dogs, as they can get very big (100+ lbs.)

Standard care for dogs:

One of the first questions you'll probably ask yourself is whether you should you let your working dogs sleep inside. This depends on what dogs you are working with, and for what purpose. If you are keeping them mostly as herding animals, and you confine your herd at night and don't need dogs to protect against predators, then they can go in a garage, for example. But if your livestock is going to be exposed to coyotes, hawks, etc., then you'll want your dogs to be around, so that you (and your herd) will feel more secure.

Dogs require core vaccines as per every state's regulations. You should give 1- or 3-year rabies shots, plus distemper/parvovirus (also 1- or 3-year). The latter is not state mandated in TN, but is a very common one that protects against contagious diseases (especially as puppies).

Situational vaccines: Bordatella (for kennel cough), Lyme Disease and Leptospirosis.

Dogs also need protection against external parasites like fleas and ticks, and internal ones like heartworms, roundworms, hookworms, and whipworms. Heartworms are mosquito-borne parasites and have become a big problem in TN, especially after Hurricane Katrina. After Katrina, many animals from Louisiana, where they were routinely exposed to heartworms, were fostered to Tennessee, providing a local "animal reservoir" for infection. This pool of infected animals then allowed local mosquitoes, which bit them, to spread it to uninfected dogs.

You should check for heartworms at least annually, because dogs can get sick and die if left unexamined. A drug called Heartgard Plus, administered monthly, is commonly used to protect dogs from heartworm infection. Another drug called Trifexis (also monthly) also provides excellent protection against heartworms. This latter drug is more expensive, but protects against a wider variety of parasites. Heartgard differs from Trifexis in that it only prevents heartworms and roundworms. Trifexis protects against heartworms, roundworms, hookworms, whipworms, and fleas (not ticks). You can give Trifexis with a supplemental flea and tick protection, and the extra flea prevention will not be a problem, as it will be a completely different mode of action.

In addition to monthly treatment for heartworms, you should also ask your vet to check fecal samples for intestinal parasites, every 6 months.

Advantage Multi is a topical medicine for fleas and ticks, with a very different mode of action than the previous two medicines. When applied to the skin, it goes into the blood, so when a flea or tick bites, its going to be killed automatically. Trifexis, on the other hand, actually goes into the subcutaneous layers of the skin after the dog has ingested it, and this prevents the fleas from even wanting to bite (thereby it works as a repellant).

Any of the ingestion methods are going to be completely different in mode of action from any topical methods, although much of the time the end result (killing of adult fleas, repellant action, etc.) can be the same.

Getting dogs spayed or neutered will not only prevent unwanted pregnancy, but can also prevent against certain sex-linked cancers. Studies are showing that animals spayed before three years can reduce the chance of ovarian and uterine cancers, and (if neutered) prostate and testicular cancers.

Vets always recommend spaying/neutering unless you know you would like to breed the animal (which can be another source of farm income, BTW) at 6 months or older.

On the diet front, raw meat, and/or a meat only diet is not generally thought to be a good thing for your dog. Dogs are omnivores and should NOT be placed on a meat-only diet. They shouldn't get too many grains, as this can lead to obesity and diabetes, but veggies are necessary in appropriate quantities. They need a balanced diet and they can get digestive and urinary problems with a meat only diet. In addition, any parasites etc. that are removed by cooking are in the meat, and can infect your dogs.

Animals, like people, are living so much longer now, largely due to better care, that the end result of most dog lives is now some form of cancer (as it is in people). However, cancer treatments in animals, as in people, have made great strides, which may be something to consider if faced with this issue, especially in a younger dog.

Cats:

Generally, cats require less maintenance than dogs. Breed specificity doesn't really matter for an outdoor farm cat. Cats are a huge benefit to any farm, culling pests such as rats, mice, voles, moles, etc. and even reptiles (e.g. snakes). They may go after birds, which, depending on your point of view, can be a good or bad thing.

Cats really like the freedom of a large property that a farm provides, and don't need much domestication. They will not really want to come indoors, but do appreciate the occasional scratch behind the ears, and will often bring you "presents" or trophies of their kills to show off to you (think of this as them paying "rent.")

It is important to mention though, that with their predation skills, you do need to be careful when cats are around certain other animals like chickens, and/or any animals that are smaller than them. Like many predators, cats tend to prey on animals smaller than themselves, so do be attentive about the access your cats may have to animals of this type on your farm.

Although you can teach a cat (stubbornly) the difference between what needs to be hunted, and does not, though this will take (lots) of time. And yes, this effort is literally a lot like herding cats!

Similarly to dogs, the standard care for cats includes state-mandated regulations of your state. Rabies is a required vaccine. Vaccinations against pathogens of the upper respiratory tract, while not required in Tennessee, are highly recommended. In addition, you should realize that your barn cats will spend 50-100% of their time outdoors. Any cat that spends a significant amount of time outdoors needs to be vaccinated for feline leukemia, and you want to test them before the vaccination to ensure they don't already have it. This is essentially a lifelong disease, similar to our leukemia in its disease process, but unlike human leukemia feline leukemia is contagious, and if unvaccinated, cats will pass it to each other, so preventing it is very important.

The internal and external parasites of cats are very similar to those of dogs, though the doses used to eradicate them are typically lower. In addition, several preventatives used in dogs are toxic to cats, so it's important to get specific feline prevention. There is a feline Heartgard and a topical Revolution to treat heartworms in cats, as well as several other feline-specific medications for various internal and external parasites.

Heartworms in cats are a lot less common than in dogs, but if they contract it, unlike dogs there is no treatment, and it will be ultimately fatal. Therefore it is important to try and get them on some kind of prevention, despite being less prevalent, because after one mosquito bite, that could be it.

The predatory behavior of cats increases the likelihood they will ingest any intestinal parasites harbored by the rodents (or other prey) they eat. So you'd probably want to have them on some sort of monthly de-wormer, or have them de-wormed every 6 months to a year. Worm transmission from cat to human can occur, so this activity is not only for their health, but also especially important if you plan to host many people on your farm, especially kids, who can, and do, get into *everything* and then put their fingers into eyes, mouths, etc.

Felines need to be spayed or neutered as well. They will proliferate very quickly if they are not, as cats can have 2-3 litters a year, and 8-12 babies at a time. Then, whereas before you had one cat, all of a sudden you have like, 60, which is not a "zero to sixty" statistic you really want, believe me!

If this happens, you'll then have feral cats running around, which you won't want to feed, and they are proliferating too, and it just gets to be a bit ugly far too quickly. Cats are the only species that we have domesticated who can go back to their feral state even after domestication.

Horses:

Your planned use of equine animals will determine whether

you'll use them as working livestock or as companions. Costs for a horse are very high. This is not just due to their purchase price, but because their feeding, medical care, and maintenance is also expensive. Cleanliness is another consideration, because you have to ensure stalls are clear of manure and flies. Stall safety, tack and hoof care are very important too.

Leigh tracked her horse expense as $16,000 per year for two horses. They were given "free" horses (if you don't think there is any such thing as a free lunch, then there REALLY isn't any such thing as a free horse). You may, in fact, really want to look that gift horse right in the mouth and say no thanks.

The 16K covered a trailer, saddles and tack, trainer fees, farrier fees, hay, feed and last but certainly not least (expensive that is), were the Vet bills. Thoroughbred horses tend to have sensitive stomachs and we had a lot of "tummy aches". Farriers had to come out every six weeks and the trainer was a weekly expense.

The horses were retired thoroughbreds (race horses), and we wanted to make them into "trail ride" horses. Farriers had to come out every six weeks. That's why in vet school, there's like the small animals, and then, not just large animals, but horses (equines).

Horses are big, powerful, and fun animals, and also very smart and friendly, but they are expensive.

Is a tractor or a working horse more economical?

Allison ran some numbers and came up with this analysis: One tractor is definitely enough to work 25 acres. A conservative rule is that you need two horses for every 25 acres. A good tractor costs about $15K, and a good young working horse is going to cost about $8K. If you have 25 acres, though, you will of course need two, so you are already a little bit more expensive just starting out on purchase cost.

Tractors save you on time and labor costs, but increase your fuel and energy costs. Horses will decrease energy costs, but will increase your labor and time, especially in the beginning until you have trained them properly. Tractors can be traded in often as late as 15 years, and you can still get about $5K for that vehicle, depending on its condition. When horses are older, also about 15 years, you can sell them too, but will only get about $1K each (they will not be working, so are at this point not going to contribute to revenue).

Costs for a tractor end up being much less than for a horse, but you have to decide what is best for you, and you can't pet a tractor (well, you could, but it won't love you back).

So assuming you'll probably want a working horse on your farm, and not a pet, we thought we'd give some information on a few of the working breeds. Most working breeds are draft horses (16-18 hands- height at the withers) and need extra girth and muscle to do the work, like these:

Belgian: These horses can pull a LOT of weight. They are usually lighter colored, with hooves the size of dinner plates (don't get stepped on). Belgians have broader heads and muzzles. They are very docile, and probably best when hauling or being driven. They work well in teams.

Percheron: These are very pretty and are another very tall breed, known for their amazing stamina. Percherons are great working horses, want to work, very intelligent, want to please you, and they love what they do.

Shire Horse: Think a thicker shaggier Clydesdale. Originally from Ireland, Shires are used in the US quite a bit, and are the breed with the record for most weight being pulled. They have broad backs, wide, thick chests, and are able to haul just about anything. These are often the horses you see when you visit an Amish farm.

Recreational breeds (trail riding, etc.): You are not going to get much working input around the farm from these, or any offset of cost.

Quarter Horse: This is the most popular breed in the US, and is a compact (14-16 hands), muscular and versatile breed, that is a great option for beginning riders.

American Standardbred: These are faster and more agile than the Quarters, and more suitable for accomplished riders.

Appaloosa: Very distinct coat color. Slim with a lean back, fast and agile.

Arabian: These have a very distinct look, dished profile on their nose, very lean, very fast. Arabians are affectionate, but also highly energetic and high-strung. They are great for long distances because they have all that stamina/energy. But you need to know what you are doing around horses to be able to handle them. If they bond with you, it's a bond for life.

Paso Fino: Best for rough terrain, good choice for a trail rider. Slight and elegant build, with a very specific gait.

Thoroughbred: (Remember! Expenses of $16,000 dollars!!!) These are beautiful, tall horses. "Thoroughbred" is actually a breed name. Very spirited breed, better for experienced riders, known for their speed and stamina, long legs, and lean body.

Standard care for horses is a little different from dogs and cats, as there are more state-mandated vaccines, including: Rabies, Tetanus, West Nile virus (mosquito-borne), EEE and WEE (Eastern and Western Equine Encephalitis, respectively). The latter are reportable, quarantineable, diseases with low survival rates, so the vaccine is very important.

In addition to the required vaccines, it may be a good idea to vaccinate horses with "risk-based" vaccines that protect against EHV (Equine Herpes Virus), and Equine Influenza. These are not mandatory in Tennessee.

The *Coggins Test* is also important to check for infectious equine anemia. This is a highly contagious, highly infectious disease, which can spread like wildfire. Everything is online via the federal regulations.

The main equine ectoparasites are flies and ticks, stable flies, and horse flies; hygiene plays a big role in controlling these. As with other animals, prevention of internal parasites is also important with horses.

Spaying and neutering can be more up to the owner with horses. This is probably a good practice if you aren't planning on breeding them, but not as high a correlation with certain cancer types as there is with dogs.

The biggest medical problems with horses are laminitis and colic. **Laminitis** is when the little leaflets in the hoof become detached from the hoof wall, and is very painful. Bones end up getting displaced, and can go through the hoof wall. It's basically like losing a fingernail suddenly and then walking on that newly exposed skin. Not really reversible, and not much you can do. There are many causes, but is typically caused by bacteria, damage and injury in general. Laminitis is a main reason why horses are shoed. It is very important to clean their hooves out very well.

You can get soft, cushiony stockings for their feet, that will help their pain a little, but the main thing is to prevent them from going septic. Bacteria will get into the blood stream and the horse will go into shock. If you get past that, they can be lame, and you can control the pain, but most people with a horse on a farm do not deal with lame horses, so they are often put down as a result.

Colic is a very generalized term for just about any kind of stomach pain in horses (or babies!). It may seem sometimes that you can just look at a horse and it gets colic. This condition apparently occurs for almost any reason, which is why it is important to immediately confer with your vet about any signs you may notice, like kicking at the stomach, rolling, biting at the rear, sweating, fever, lying on their side, not getting up, etc.

Colic can be due to an obstruction, the intestines being twisted around each other, blood being cut off, etc. Intervention is nearly always required as colic will not go away on its own, and surgery is frequently required (and will be expensive). Vets will try almost anything before surgery, because most of the time when they have colic, they're going to have it again, so if you can get rid of it with some antibiotics and pain meds, that's the first thing tried, but if they have to do surgery, you're looking at about $10-20K.

Remember: if they're walking funny, it's laminitis, if they are rolling around in discomfort, its probably colic.

Cattle:

Raising animals on pasture means feeding them primarily or solely grass growing in the field. In this method of raising animals, the farmer rotates the grazing area for the animals by moving them regularly (how often this rotation occurs depends on the animal and the size of the grazing area). Meat from such animals is called "grass-fed," "pastured," or "pasture-raised."

Many different livestock can be raised this way: beef, chicken, rabbits, sheep, and goats, to name a few.

But as a small farmer considering pasture-raised animals vs. the conventional way of feeding them grain, you might wonder: why should I do this? What are the benefits to me as a farmer? How about to the animals or the buyer? Will I have a market for this meat? Will consumers care? Does it taste different?

It turns out that pasture-raised meat and dairy actually has naturally occurring healthy properties

Products from pasture-raised, grass-fed animals contain higher amounts of certain beneficial nutrients, such as: vitamin E, beta-carotene, conjugated linoleic acid (CLA), and omega-3 fatty acids, which are antioxidants and/or vitamins that our bodies need. In humans, CLA is associated with a lower incidence of tumors and certain cancers (including breast cancer).

Omega-3 fatty acids have anti-inflammatory properties, which can be helpful in the prevention of heart disease, and, as humans don't eat grass, are found naturally in relatively high amounts in fish, seafood and algae. Omega-6 and Omega-3 fatty acids usually occur together in different ratios, with a higher ratio of Omega-3 being more desirable. Most humans get too much Omega-6, which is high in grain-fed animals, and not enough Omega-3 (higher in grass-fed). People take Omega-3 supplements to help combat cancer, asthma, obesity, depression, and many other inflammatory conditions.

The vitamin E in grass-fed meat has the benefits of Vitamin E from any other source, and also helps keep meat from spoiling as quickly.

Does grass-fed meat taste better?

Many people believe that pasture-fed meat tastes better, and at least one study, which showed that pastured rabbits produced tastier and more tender meat, seems to support this.

Frequent anecdotal reports from farmers and consumers support the idea that grass-fed meat just plain tastes better. The beef from grass-fed cows is often leaner overall, and the fat that is there is, again, higher in Omega-3. Even though it has less fat and marbling, it is still very tender.

Grass-Fed Meat may be safer

Cornell University and the USDA have done research on the types of E. coli, (a potentially pathogenic bacteria), found in the stomachs of grass-fed versus grain-fed beef cattle. Grain-fed beef has a higher concentration of acid-resistant E. coli. This can be a concern because the acid resistance allows the bacteria to survive the human stomach environment and cause food poisoning.

Never mind comparing mass-produced, grain-fed animals to small-scale grass-fed animals in terms of how they are raised and the way conditions on a small farm are often more sanitary due to lack of overcrowding.

Pastured Animals are Better Treated, and Probably Healthier:

Cattle are meant to roam on grasses and eat them. Turkeys and chickens are meant to roam, forage for bugs, and eat plants. Rabbits eat grass. Sheep, obviously, eat grass. When animals are allowed to pasture, they live a life more in tune with their natural inclinations, the life they are genetically programmed to thrive living.

This results in fewer health problems for the farmer. Dairy cows raised on grass generally have fewer foot problems. They also have lower rates of acidosis. Beef cattle raised on grass have fewer liver lesions. In general, pastured animals require fewer antibiotics and less medical intervention.

Grass-Fed Animals Are More Economical to Raise

What could be more economical than *not* buying feed? When you're able to raise animals on grass, you save on buying grain. Even if you grow hay for your animals to eat during winter, it is still less expensive than confinement feeding.

Grass-Fed Animals Benefit the Environment

You can't get more local than your animals eating what grows on the ground in front of them. Plus, the natural grasses that make up pasture are much better for the environment, from a CO_2 perspective, than tilled crops. The plants remove CO_2 from the air during photosynthesis. Without having to use oil-powered machinery to harvest feed, spread manure, or truck grain, the environment benefits. Growing pasture grasses is much more friendly to the soil than growing and harvesting grain crops.

Yes, Customers Understand the Benefits:

More and more, consumers are asking for grass-fed products. They have learned or read about the benefits described above, and they want this healthier, more environmentally sustainable meat! You should definitely do your market research and build a business plan, if this is an avenue you want to explore, but the demand for grass-fed products is definitely increasing.

Finally, and perhaps most importantly for the purposes of this book, grass feeding, for many of the reasons listed above, is a more consistently SUSTAINABLE farming method than grain feeding. So yes, we would thoroughly endorse this feeding method as being consistent with sustainable farming practice.

Beef vs. Dairy

To be honest, raising beef or dairy cattle is probably not very cost effective for smaller farms, if you only have two or three animals. It's predominantly the larger production farms/ranches that make the most money.

But if you want the cows for personal meat or dairy consumption, then that can be a totally viable option. Just bear in mind, on the beef side especially, that if you are a small operation with only a few animals, it might become emotionally difficult for you to slaughter them (especially if you name them) when compared to the large beef operations, which are much more impersonal.

Beef Breeds:

Angus: This is the most popular "carcass breed" that is out there (I know, kind of a grim term, right?) These cattle are naturally "polled" (don't have horns). They come in black and red varieties, are very hardy in almost any environment, good-natured, docile and easy to handle, which is good because beef breeds can be a little spirited compared to dairy breeds. (The latter are handled all the time, and so are used to constant contact with humans).

Charolais: These are *huge* animals. The Charolais has a long body, and is extremely muscular, with heavy-muscled loins and haunches. They are typically white with pink skin. They are also fairly easy to manage and also adaptable to a wide range of environments (except extreme ones, like, you know, frozen tundra, which may not be the best place to start a sustainable farm anyway. Just saying).

Hereford: This is probably the second most popular breed in the US, after the Angus. They have to have white faces, and can be any color after that. They are known for being really docile, and also for maturing quickly, which is important in the beef field because you want to get a return on that feeding investment as soon as possible.

Gelbvieh: This breed is not well known, but is a pretty moderate one: medium size, average muscling, and have sweet, quiet dispositions. They are also easy to take care of.

Limousin: (Yes, really, that's its name). And yes, this will be a large animal. Hailing from France originally, they have a long body, short neck and muzzle, and a very lean carcass. Very large frame (strong bones) with lean meat (More bone density typically equals less fat, less bone, relatively speaking, means higher fat content.) So an Angus, which is not as big as a Limousine, will have more marbling.

Simmental: This is another white-faced animal. However, too much white around the eyes can lead to eye cancer, as there is no protective pigmentation in the vicinity. So Simmentals are bred to have pigment around the eyes, to help mitigate this issues. With lean carcasses, Simmentals have been bred to be huge, easy to take care of, and good-natured, because the ones that aren't you won't want to keep around. All the breeds are similar in that sense.

Dairy Breeds:

Dairy cattle are typically a little more docile than their beef counterparts (maybe they know they aren't going to be killed and eaten?) Another general rule about dairy is that a higher protein and butterfat content, usually translates into more sought after milk, commanding higher prices. But the breeds that make the most protein typically don't make as much milk, which offsets total revenue somewhat.

Ayreshire: These are red and white, and speckled. Medium sized to strong and rugged, they easily adapt as well. They are bred to reduce foot and leg problems, and have fewer problems in their feet and legs than some other breeds. This is a moderate butterfat breed. One of the things you consider when thinking of starting a dairy herd, is the protein and butterfat ratios, so each breed will have a different ratio of butterfat (which comes out in the supermarket as your 2%, 1%, etc.)

Brown Swiss: These are usually light in color, with cream muzzles and dark noses. Strong and well balanced, they have fewer problems calving, are great cheese makers, with high protein and high butterfat. This is a good all around dairy cow.

Holstein: A California cow, this is the most common dairy cow in the US. Most commonly black and white, they can also be red and white. Holsteins are easily adaptable, best for low cost management, they can forage, are easy to handle, and are great animals. Low input for the amount of output that you get.

Jersey: These are probably the second most popular US breed, and provide milk at lower cost than most breeds, have higher protein and BF, so you can sell for a higher price as well. Probably don't make as much quantity of milk as other breeds with lower protein milk.

Do people eat dairy cows for their beef? After a cow's milk production it's utility ends, and some people will then use the cow for its beef. Grass fed dairy cattle taste fine, but the meat will not be as highly marbled and tender as the beef you buy at the grocery store. Plus, as they tend to be older animals, you will have lot of bone as well, and a fair amount of fat around the various cuts (as this is what gives milk its fat content).

Dairy cattle are much smaller than beef cattle, as they are bred for milk production (800 lbs. vs. 1500 lbs. for beef cattle).

Standard Care of Cattle:

Care is pretty much the same for both beef and dairy cattle. Various vaccines are required, for diseases with very long names, against viruses specific to cattle. Dairy cattle are typically housed in stalls, and then let out to feed, etc., so sanitation and ventilation of the barn is very important.

Also, as in other animals, cattle need protection against flies and ticks, and intestinal parasites. Cows are a bit easier to administer to, as you don't have to ensure, for instance, that they ingest a Heartworm pill, you can either just inject it, or apply in a pour on, which is literally poured over the back of the animal.

Cattle are not usually spayed or neutered, because so much of the cattle husbandry is based on breeding and continuing on the lines.

Good nutrition is vital. Any kind of ruminant can bloat easily, so non-contaminated feed with no mold from a reliable source is very important.

Milk production in cattle is initiated through breeding, either through artificial insemination, or via a breeding bull that comes in as a "stud." They generate milk while they are pregnant, and you make it continue by the massaging motion of milking around feeding time. Cows are easily trained to come to eat at specific times of the day (can sound a horn every time you feed them, or hey, even ring a cowbell, what a concept). A good dairy cow can usually provide milk about 300 days of the year. The rest of the time when they aren't, it's usually because they are about to have a baby. When the cow calves, they will still provide milk, but you usually let her feed her baby at this time for about 2 months, then you just continue milking the mom after the calf is weaned.

Dairy cattle get very uncomfortable if you don't milk them, because their udders get so full, and there is a great deal of nerve stimulation down there. The action of milking continues the hormone response of continued oxytocin production, which is instrumental in milk production, and they must be fed a whole lot while they are milking as a proper, nutrient rich diet also helps produce the milk.

The combination of nutrition, the hormone production/timing around pregnancy, and giving milk to the baby, as well as the physical massage of the teats (which mimics the calf trying to latch on and suckle milk), all combine to perpetuate milk production in those breeds which have been bred for the purpose.

A cow will continue to produce milk for several months after her calf is weaned, then you need to breed them again, so you have to pay attention to when the cow is in oestrus (heat). Sometimes, as the cow ages, you might want to give them a season off, but it's pretty continuous. Artificial insemination is more expensive than having a bull, but you have better success rates.

You don't have to keep the babies if you don't want to (you can sell them to other dairy farmers, e.g.) but you may also want to keep them to become milkers on your farm. After their "milking career" is over, some people keep their dairy cows as pets, because they are very sweet, but just bear in mind that there is nonfinancial advantage to doing this, as they will no longer be offsetting the cost of their keep through milk production.

Dairy cows mature fairly early, and you can usually start breeding around eight to ten months, so that you are beginning to see a return on that investment fairly soon after you start to house them.

Having dairy cattle is a 24/7, 365 days/year, dedicated job. You (or someone else) HAVE to be there for both milkings, which are usually roughly 12 hours apart, every single day, so you will see a lot of dairy farmers burn out. There is a little wriggle room with feeding times, but not much, some people feed at 6 and 6, others at 4 and 4.

Either way, you are getting up pretty early if you want to go down this road.

That being said, you will enjoy your very own creamy milk, butter and cheese, which will taste far better than anything you will buy at the supermarket, and you may be able to make a small income from the sale of these items as well.

Despite their need to release milk, cows are not very accepting of calves that are not theirs, and calves who mix up their Moms will often get a rude awakening, usually in the form of a swift kick, if they try to approach the wrong udder.

Milking your cow:

How, exactly, do you do this process if you never have before?

Obviously, it's ideal to watch and learn in person, from a dairy farmer, and to have some chances to practice first. But if you can't, don't worry. You can figure this out on your own.

Generally speaking, if you can milk by hand, this is the best way for a small operation. A milking machine won't save time, because it takes time to set it up and clean it. But if your hands aren't strong enough or you have health problems that preclude hand milking, by all means use a milking machine.

Keeping your hands, the equipment, and the cow's udder very clean will help prevent bacteria from infesting your milk.

Before you begin, set up a bucket with fresh, warm water, disinfectant and a cloth. Brush the side of the cow you'll milk on. Set up your stool and use the cloth and warm water and disinfectant to wash the cow's udder. This action simulates a calf stimulating the udder and helps the cow "let down " its milk. That means her milk will flow from the upper part of the udder into the teat.

Letdown lasts only about ten minutes, during which time you

will milk the teats.

You start by gently squeezing the top of the teat with your thumb and forefinger. Then, with your fingers resting along the teat, squeeze each one closed in turn, all the way down until you reach the end of the teat. Release all your fingers, to allow the teat to fill up again with milk, and then repeat.

Once you get into a rhythm, you can work two teats at a time, alternating first one and then the other.

Also, with the first stream from each teat, squeeze it onto the floor or into a separate cup so you can observe it first. It should look clean and be the proper color: no clots, lumps or blood. This is also a generally good hygiene practice, as the first stream of milk is most likely to contain any pathogenic bacteria.

As the flow slows down, reduce your milking to one teat at a time, using the other hand to gently massage the upper part of the udder. You will want to ensure that you get all the milk out of the udder, to prevent an infection called mastitis.

Once the milk is in the bucket, you must cool and strain it quickly. You can buy a commercial milk strainer, or pour the milk through at least four layers of clean cheesecloth, or dishtowels laid in a clean colander over a bowl.

You can pasteurize the milk if you want, as well: before cooling, but after straining it. Home milk pasteurization machines can be purchased locally or online, or you can use a stovetop method. You can also make butter with the milk fat.

Common Health Issues with Cattle:

Mastitis: Mastitis can happen in beef cattle, but is less frequent, because mainly in beef you are keeping the males, and in dairy you are keeping the females, and mastitis most frequently is due to sanitation problems during milking. You will need to sanitize each udder before you start milking, and then use gloves, as we humans have commensal (harmless, but present) bacteria all over our skin that can infect the cow, traveling up their teat to cause infection in the teat and udder, with pus production and other unpleasant side effects.

You have to continue milking a cow even if it has mastitis, but the milk that you get has to be thrown out, not only due to the potential for bacteria, but because it will also house all those inflammation processes in it. The good news is that any milk that you drink is not going to have come from a cow with mastitis.

Lameness: This is not as bad as laminitis in horses, but cows can pick up an infection which causes them to hobble around, usually cured by footbath. Cows often poop while they are milking (don't ever wear nice clothes while doing this chore), and stand in it until the milking is over. So typically dairy cattle are called in, milked first, and then if they need one, are given a footbath on the way back, out into pasture.

Forage and Friends:

Forage acreage per cow is usually about 2-5 acres per animal. White clover is a big cause of bloat, so you'd like to have other grasses like alfalfa or fescue to supplement this. One cow is likely sufficient to provide dairy products for a family for much of the year. Two milkings a day will usually yield 1-2 liters a day, so if you want to drink a lot of milk, and make cheese, and butter as well, you might want to have two cows. This can also be good for the cows from an emotional/social standpoint. It's a dairy legend, but probably true, that happy cows give more and better milk.

Having two Holsteins together, for example, can be good for them. Cows, particularly dairy cattle, are very social animals. Those cow commercials are true; cows have best friends, and gossip together. Having one cow won't make that one upset or depressed, but having others around would likely make them happier, which could also positively impact their milk production.

But you don't even need another cow; it can be any sort of friendly sociable animal like a herding dog, for instance. There are many, many stories of these wonderful friendships that develop between animals of completely different species.

Goats:

Goats can be great animals to add to your farm. They're easy to handle and produce lots of delicious and healthful milk as well as low-fat meat. Plus, goat manure makes great fertilizer.

Should You Raise Goats?

One doe will produce 90 quarts of fresh milk every month for 10 months of the year, with two months off right before she gives birth. That said, goats are really social and you can't keep just one doe - you'll need to keep two goats, a doe and a wether, or two does, at a minimum, so they don't get lonely.

Each castrated male goat, or "meat wether," will produce 25 to 40 pounds of meat. And each bred doe will give birth to, at minimum, one kid annually.

Goats don't need fussy housing, but they do require some serious fencing to keep them where they belong. They will graze pasture but are great browsers, who will eat bushes and other brush. Dairy goats will require some hay and commercial goat feed too though, so you'll need to be prepared to feed them. Meat goats do well on just hay and browsing, unless they're nursing or growing kids.

Raising Goats for Milk or Meat:

Like cattle, goats can be used for either milk or meat production. They can also be used for wool and hair production, although because these breed types have such thick coats, most farmers in Tennessee, where it can get very hot in the summer, still mostly use sheep for this latter purpose.

Goat meat is not a typical staple in most of Tennessee, and is not commonplace in the US in general. But there is a demand for it from certain religious and cultural groups who predominantly eat it, and it can be a profitable niche if you find the right market. There is in fact such a demand that goat meat must be imported into the US every year. It's fairly easy to keep dairy goats and raise the bucks for meat, since you have to breed your does to keep them in milk and roughly half of all kids are male. However, the Boer is the main meat breed in the US, primarily raised for meat not milk. Another option is to breed your milking goats to Boers or another meat breed to produce crossbred kids for meat, while still keeping does for milk.

Housing and Fencing Goats:

Goat housing is simple: just keep them dry and draft-free and they are happy. A three-sided structure is enough for mild climates. It's helpful to have a small stall for isolating a sick or injured goat or for a pregnant goat to give birth. Packed dirt will suffice for a floor in the goat house, but it should be covered with a thick layer of bedding: wood shavings (not cedar), straw, or waste hay. Since hay is goats' primary food and they tend to waste up to one-third of it, you can pitch the waste hay into the bedding area each day, saving money. Keep bedding clean and dry, spreading new layers on top and removing and replacing all of it as needed.

Fencing is a little more complex. Goats need a very strong fence that they can't climb over, knock down or otherwise escape from. If there is so much as a tiny hole, they will find a way to get out. They use their lips to explore their world, so if a gate latch is loose, they can wiggle it open with their lips and escape. They also chew almost everything - rope, electrical wiring, and so on, are all fair game. And goats can jump and climb. Your goat house should have a climbing-proof roof.

High-tensile, smooth electrified wire is ideal if you want to take an existing fence and make it goat-proof. You can use a nonelectric fence at least four feet high, five feet for active breeds like Nubians. You should brace the corners and gates on the outside so the goats can't climb up the braces. You can use wooden fencing, stock panels, or chain-link fence, or you can combine a wooden rail fence with woven wire.

Feeding Goats:

As mentioned, goats can be pastured on grass, or browse in the woods, eating shrubs and young trees. It's important to rotate goats to new pasture so that they graze it evenly and don't foul it up, which can lead to a buildup of parasites.

Goats require additional hay even when they have pasture, as they can't eat all fresh grass. You can feed them as much as they desire. Young goats and pregnant or milk-producing does require some goat "concentrate," or goat chow.

True to stereotype, goats will eat garbage, and could potentially eat the tin can they find lying around, but it won't get any nutrients from it. They will clear the brush and clear your garbage, but you do want to ensure they are getting good nutrition as well.

One thing you need to watch out for is if you have hemlock on your property, goats will eat it and it will kill them. They will pretty much eat anything, including shirts (while being worn), hair (while on your head), and any stuff you have on your hair.

Goats are super fun to have around the farm, as they tend to have very definite personalities. They are typically frisky and energetic, and have a great ability to forage and adapt to almost any environment. They are also easy to manage, and are very low maintenance. We have three goats on our property. We had more, but the coyotes sadly killed all the babies one year and we haven't had the heart to start another herd.

Donkeys and mules are often pastured with other livestock, as they are an amazing defense against coyotes. Llamas are interestingly also good as anti-predator animals. We are investigating the possibility of fostering a donkey. They could protect any future kid goats and the feed can be tax-deductible... a win-win.

Meat Breeds:

Boer: We have Boer-mix goats. These can grow to be very large (recall how beef cattle tend to have large bodies as well). Boer goats tend to have full white bodies, with darker heads, and long droopy ears. Just as an aside, it can sometimes be hard to tell goats and sheep apart. Goats' tails go up, and wag upright, while sheep tails hang down. Goat tails are also typically longer, and sheep tails are what we call "docked." This is because since they hang down they can get a lot of fecal matter on it, so their tails are cut at a very young age to prevent this.

Boer goats are probably the most popular goat-meat breed in the world, not just in the US. They have a really fast growth rate, and high fertility, which is good both in terms of turnaround of investment and if you suffer herd culling from predators. The quality of the meat is typically very high and like many goats these have an increased resistance to disease. Vaccinating your goats is still optimal, but there is a lower risk of them getting sick than is the case with other animals such as horses and cows.

Goats are usually friendly, although they can be more territorial if they have a lot of kids around, in which case take a branch with you and smack them on the head if they get too belligerent. This might sound a little mean, but you have to show a goat who is boss, and, in their eyes, be the goat that isn't backing down.

Kiko: These are pretty common in Tennessee. Generally very large-framed, all white, hardy and able to thrive under poor conditions, the Kiko was developed in New Zealand and brought to the US in the 1990s. They are a bit friskier than the Boers, and are known for substantial weight gain without any supplemental feeding. If you have a lot of range available, Kikos may be a more economical breed than Boers for you to raise.

Spanish: Before Boer goats became popular in the US in the late

1980s, Spanish goats were the standard meat-goat breed, especially in the South. They are so named because they are descended from goats first introduced to the Americas by Spanish explorers. They were originally bred for brush and pasture maintenance, but then due to selection they became mixed with other breeds to become a meat breed. They're medium-sized and lanky, mostly short-haired, and come in all colors. They don't need a lot of supplemental feeding and can breed out of season. This means a higher production of kids (like, everywhere). They have long, often twisty horns.

Dairy Breeds:

The three most popular dairy goat breeds (though there are others) in the US are the La Mancha, Nubian, and Toggenburg.

La Mancha: These are friendly goats that come in a variety of colors and patterns, La Manchas usually have small ears (sometimes so small as to be unnoticeable) of two types: gopher ears, small and rounded, or slightly larger ears, shorter than two inches, that some people call "elf ears."

This is one of the smaller dairy breeds, but they tend to be very high milk producers. They are very popular in Middle Tennessee, and you'll find them at many county fairs.

Nubian: Nubian goats are one of the most popular dairy breeds in the world, and the most popular American dairy breed. With their floppy, long ears and rounded, convex noses (called "Roman" noses), they are large goats producing a rich milk high in butterfat. Goat-cheese makers often choose Nubian milk because of this quality. They don't produce the same volume of milk as the La Manchas, but they're sometimes called "the Jerseys of the dairy goat world," because like Jersey cows, they produce a milk so high in protein and butterfat.

One thing to be aware of that Nubians can be very loud, and they have a distinctive cry that may annoy your neighbors. They are also not quite as manageable as other more docile breeds.**Toggenberg:** Toggenburg goats, or Toggs, as they are sometimes called, are a very sweet-tempered, medium-sized breed, coming in a variety of colors: from light brown to chocolate. They are known for having attractive markings such as white-sided tails, white muzzles, white ears, and two stripes down the face. They are one of the only dairy breeds with erect ears, and tend to be a little shaggier than the other more straight-coated breeds. Spirited and playful, Toggs are average milk volume producers (lower than La Manchas, for instance), and their milk is lower fat than the Nubians. But they have extra long lactation periods, which means they provide milk for more days in the year.

Goat milk is very different than any kind of cow's milk. It's a different, stronger flavor, thickness and texture. Feta and goat cheeses are made from goat's milk, as is the white queso dip you see at many Mexican restaurants.

The full pasteurization process (for both cattle and goats) is very involved and beyond the scope of this book. It is possible to drink unpasteurized milk, but its important to remember that there is a risk of bacterial contamination (from bacteria already present in the milk), which can lead to infection of us humans if you do this.

"Fun" Breeds:

Pygmy Goats: Pygmy goats are highly domesticated and are mostly pets, but they are actually officially listed as meat goats because they have a compact and meaty body and are fertile out of season. They are very energetic, and very entertaining to watch, and a lot of fun. They do tend to poop when and where they want, but the upside is their poop is pellet-like, and very easy to clean up.

Tennessee Fainting Goats: Tennessee Fainting goats are, in fact, from Tennessee and are also call myotonic goats, Nervous goats, Wooden goats or Stiff Leg goats.

When startled, these goats go rigid and "faint" or fall down. This is actually a painless genetic disorder that has been intentionally perpetuated by breeding. Originally, the genetic disorder would turn up in large herds and the poor goat would be the "fall guy" when the herd was attacked by a predator. So the goats were bred for this purpose, to protect the rest of the herd. Now they are a specialty breed that is used strictly for enjoyment and companionship.

If you have these goats, you do need to keep them confined, because they are easy prey for predators (fainting and falling down is not a great survival strategy when the coyotes are coming). Myotonic goats are hardy, fertile, and have a long breeding season.

Standard Care of Goats:

Despite their general hardiness, goats can be susceptible to certain strains of *Clostridium* bacteria, and also tetanus and there are core vaccines for these.

As with other animals, you will need to worry about flies and ticks, as well as intestinal parasites. The number one intestinal parasite of goats is called *Haemoncus contortus*, otherwise known as the Barber pole worm. This is an almost ubiquitous worm that is found in almost every goat, and which can be fatal.

H. contortus is a voracious bloodsucker that causes severe anemia, which will be observable by color changes in the mucus membranes around the eye. The FAMACHA@ eye color chart has been developed so that goat producers can observe goat's symptoms for possible infestation by parasites. (FAMACHA stands for "Faffa Malan's Chart," named after its developer, Dr. Faffa Malan).

FAMACHA is a system that allows farmers to easily check each goat or sheep and determine whether or not deworming is needed. In the past, entire herds were wormed on a monthly schedule. But as in the case with overuse of antibiotics in humans, this led to a high percentage of the Barber Pole worm population becoming resistant to the antihelminthic (de-wormer medicine). As more of the worms that were susceptible to the anti-helminthic medicines were killed, the only ones left to mate with each other were de-wormer resistant worms. This has led to a sort of "Super Barber Pole Worm" population.

Why use FAMACHA?

Since the problem is an anthelmintic resistant worm population, the answer seemed to be to re-introduce weaker, antihelminthic-susceptible worms back into the population. To accomplish this the treatment strategy has centered on leaving the weaker worms alive unless absolutely necessary. In order to do that, although it seems counter-intuitive, dewormer is only given to those goats or sheep that are showing signs of anemia (the main symptom of barber pole worm infestation) that has reached an unsafe level.

Prevention (or perhaps more properly "mitigation") and treatment strategies have been developed; beginning with seasonal or monthly egg counts in feces and use of the FAMACHA test. These counts will identify your highest shedders (worms, not hair), and your most symptomatic animals (white mucus membranes), and then you will de-worm them. You are deliberately not trying to eliminate everything, and the goats you don't treat will tend to propagate the antihelminthic-susceptible worms.

The fecal egg counts are managed by you collecting a bag of their feces and taking it to the vet, and de-worming is accomplished by feeding the goat a liquid deworming paste that you put in their mouths, on a seasonal basis.

Special Considerations for Ruminants (Cows, Goats and Sheep):

Cows have four so-called stomach compartments: the rumen reticulum, omasum, and abomasum (or "true" stomach).

When cows eat, the food goes down the esophagus, into the rumen and reticulum, then is regurgitated back up the esophagus for them to re-chew, which makes the particle size be small enough for further digestion in the omasum and abomasum.

The Reticulum:

The reticulum traps anything that the cow should not have eaten, such as pieces of fencing, rocks and pieces of wire. The reticulum also softens the grass that has been eaten and forms small wads of cud. "Hardware disease" can happen when a ruminant swallows metal, which then gets trapped in the reticulum. Because of the cow's ongoing digestive action, sharp metal objects can then puncture the reticulum wall, then possibly the diaphragm, and even get to the heart. The vet will typically make the cow swallow a magnet, which will attract the metal, and the weight of the magnet will prevent the metal from travelling back up the reticulum, preventing puncture. This will stay there indefinitely: in case the cow swallows more metal, the magnet will trap it as well.

The Rumen:

The rumen is the largest part of the cow's stomach, holding up to 50 gallons of partially digested food at any given time. It contains enzymes that start the digestion process, breaking down the hard food and cellulose. The food may spend 15 to 48 hours in and out of the rumen being chewed, swallowed, regurgitated and swallowed again and again, before moving on to the second part of the stomach, the reticulum. This constant chewing and saliva production keeps the digestive process going, which, especially in cows, is necessary due to the length of the digestive tract and the need to keep things moving along.

The Omasum:

The omasum has many folds to filter the food, squeeze out water, and further break down the cud.

The Abomasum:

The abomasum completes the digestion process. It passes essential nutrients to the bloodstream and sends the rest through the intestines. A Displaced Abomasum can be an issue with cattle: The abomasum usually lies along the floor of the abdomen, but when it fills with gas it can travel to the top, get displaced or stuck somewhere and cause the cow a lot of pain. This will manifest a little like colic in horses, and the cow may kick and roll around. This issue typically requires surgery to be corrected, and after being pulled back the abomasum will be tacked to the side of the abdominal wall so that the displacement won't happen again (there being an 80% likelihood of it happening again if it happens once).

The causes of a displaced abomasum are many and varied. If the cow rolls around the abomasum can flop over, if they have trauma, like going through a chute and it doesn't fit, or perhaps birthing (a difficult birth) can all cause a displaced abomasum.

Bloat: Bloat is due to an abnormal buildup of gas in the rumen (from eating the wrong things) Bloat usually happens around spring, when the grass and flower are in bloom, as most of the white flowers like white clover can cause bloat. The gas from these can usually be burped out, but if not the cow will get bloat, and may exhibit colic like symptoms again.

Withdrawal times: Withdrawal time is the USDA-mandated time given to allow vaccines and medicines to clear from the meat or milk. If you have a sick cow, for instance, and you are giving it penicillin, you will still be milking it but you will be tossing the milk away, because it will contain the antibiotic (and likely also the inflammatory processes of the disease as well as bacteria). Withdrawal times can be found online from the USDA website and you have to follow these rules to a "T."

There are some medicines, like certain steroids, that if you give cows may never clear the system, so if they go to slaughter and you are trying to sell the meat you can get into serious trouble.

Therefore before giving any vaccine, de-wormer, antibiotic, etc., you need to check the withdrawal time.

Chickens:

The Chicken, or the Egg?

Deciding the answer to this question is the critical first step, before you actually get the chicks. Consider whether you really want to raise meat birds. They're very different from egg-laying hens. You'll have a lot (usually 50 or more, although you could just raise a few) of fast-growing birds, which means a lot of poop. And perhaps the biggest question to answer is: can you handle saying goodbye in a relatively short time? Whether you slaughter them on-farm or take them to be processed, if you're a new farmer, you will need to face this reality, or be a vegetarian farmer. It's up to you, but don't agonize it after the fact: it's considered cruel to let meat birds live longer than a few months as they are heavy-breasted and can die of heart failure if they grow too big.

Some breeds can be used either for meat or for egg production. Assuming that you aren't looking to invest in a huge broiler facility, our discussion on chickens will focus mostly around how to produce fresh eggs. You may or may not want to use the chickens for meat once their laying cycle is done, but by then they are literally not spring chickens anymore, and not as tender as they might be, so you'd want to think about this too, before slaughtering your previous egg layers for meat consumption.

Should you get a rooster?

Contrary to popular misconception, you don't need a rooster for your hens to lay eggs. A rooster is needed to fertilize the eggs, to hatch them into baby chicks, but hens will lay just as many eggs whether there's a rooster around or not.

Some farmers would rather keep an all-female flock, and urban or suburban homesteaders may not have a choice, due to zoning laws that forbid roosters.

When you keep a rooster, you have to be careful about broody hens (who will sit on the eggs, hoping they will hatch), because the eggs will start developing into baby chicks if fertilized. You can use the broody hen to hatch eggs, but this involves some decision-making and supervision, so that the eggs you eat aren't the ones she's sitting on.

Some farmers prefer to have a rooster, because he does offer significant protection for the flock. He will guard against predators and sound the alert if there is any perceived danger. We prefer to have a rooster because we think the girls get along better… but that is personal preference.

Pros of Having a Rooster:

Roosters will protect their hens from predators, keeping them safe by keeping them together and sounding the alert if a predator approaches. He will also defend them bodily against an attacker!

They also complete the natural order of the flock. Chickens naturally live with males and females mixed, so you're allowing your hens to live as "normal" a life as possible with a rooster in the mix. And owners have reported that roosters will break up "hen fights," (think cat fights with feathers), find and give treats to their girls, encourage egg-laying, and even monitor the nest boxes.

Roosters are iconic farmyard animals, and they are gorgeous to look at in many cases. They also have a lot of personality (think of the terms "cock of the walk, " or "cock-a-hoop"), so they can be very entertaining and interesting creatures to have around.

You will need one if you want to naturally hatch baby chicks. My grandddaddy Parker raised natural flocks, and the roosters were good daddies to their babies and took care of the mother hen too. We choose not to hatch our own chicks and order them from a hatchery. Twenty-five chicks come in the US Mail, delivered overnight, in a small box with air holes. The boxes are different sizes, depending on what time of the year they are ordered… larger (for more air flow) in the summer, and smaller (for more warmth) in the winter.

Cons of Having a Rooster:

One of the biggest cons of having a rooster is that his presence may violate your local zoning laws. Obviously, if your city or county doesn't allow them, don't get a rooster! You're just asking for trouble.

Even if your local laws don't prohibit them, remember they can be noisy. Yes, they do crow, and yes, in the morning, and yes, at other inopportune times as well. Think of how you will like this when it happens, and also about your neighbors' reactions, especially if you live in close quarters.

Roosters can also be aggressive. They have spurs on their ankles that can break skin. You need to stay on top of "training" them that you're the BIG rooster, so they respect you, and you might want to think about it if you have small children or lots of farm visitors.

They can "wear out" hens (Ahem!). At the risk of too much information, sex between a rooster and a hen is in no way what humans would call consensual, and if you have too many roosters and too few hens (one rooster can "take care of" up to 30 hens), your hens will start to show the wear: (backs rubbed clean of feathers, for example), they'll be just plain worn out. So keep your rooster to hen ratio in the healthy zone!

How to Start Breeding Hens:

When considering purchasing chickens for your farm, there are some very professional, reputable online hatcheries that will send you chicks, and we recommend you consider buying through breeding programs such as these. We order our chicks from McMurray Hatchery based in Iowa, and their website is https://www.mcmurrayhatchery.com

Most breeders will provide certain guarantees with them (e.g. certain number of males, females etc.) but this is not 100% reliable, as sexing eggs is ridiculously difficult. You will always get a couple of roosters (which you won't want as, surprise, these don't lay eggs). Our most recent breed is a sex link chicken called Red Star. They are brown-egg layers and consistently produce an egg a day from each hen. The Hatchery guaranteed all hens, since the sex link showed the females as reddish brown chicks and the males as yellow chicks… easy to separate.

Three Main Breeding Birds:

Leghorns: This is the breed that was popularized in cartoon form on *The Bugs Bunny Road Runner Show*©. They lay moderate-sized white eggs, and are well suited for uninterrupted laying (280-300 eggs per year). They have two laying cycles and will start out slowly, and then a good layer will lay once to twice a day. Then, after 50-60 weeks, they will stop producing for a month or two, during their "molt" cycle (when they will regenerate their lost pin feathers). After the molt, they will then proceed to their second laying cycle, which is less productive. After the second molt, laying becomes sporadic.

According to the McMurray Hatchery website: "Over 45 years of scientific breeding research have gone into the development of this layer through a blending of special strains of White Leghorns. These pullets weigh about 4 lbs. at maturity, start laying at 4 1/2 to 5 months, and will continue laying 10 to 12 weeks longer than most good layers. Livability and resistance to disease are very high, and the feed to egg conversion ratio is excellent, holding down the cost of egg production. When our local farmers ask us to recommend the pullet that will lay the most eggs of top grade and size, of uniform shape, good shell, and highest interior quality, and do it on the least feed and in smallest amount of space, we suggest the Pearl."

Plymouth Rock: This bird comes in many different colors, have red earlobes, with a deep full breast and abdomen, which are great attributes for laying eggs. They live longer than other breeds, but this doesn't necessarily mean they will produce eggs longer. These birds are great in cold temperatures.

(Note: chickens are not as temperature robust as other animals, such as goats. Many breeds don't like the cold, and in cold temperatures you will likely need a heater in the coop, while when it is hot, you should probably open all the doors, and perhaps even put in a fan, as we do).

Plymouths are pretty docile, and lay large brown eggs. Egg production varies among the various subtypes of this breed, but mimics the output of the Leghorn.

The McMurray website states: "Prolific layers of brown eggs, the hens are not discouraged by cold weather. Their solid plumpness and yellow skin make a beautiful heavy roasting fowl. Their bodies are long, broad, and deep with bred-in strength and vitality."

Rhode Island Reds: This is one of the most famous and all time popular breeds of truly American chickens. Developed in the early part of this century in the state of the same name, they have maintained their reputation as a dual-purpose fowl through the years. Outstanding for their egg-production qualities, this breed has led the contests for brown egg layers time after time. No other heavy breed lays more or better eggs than the Rhode Island Reds. Baby chicks are a rusty red color and the mature birds are a variety of mahogany red.

This is definitely the most popular breed for backyard layers, which may be the type of small flock most single-family farms will have. They are very cost-effective, but our experience has shown that they are not one of the most docile, so although you will have the usual "pecking order" you may want to consider another breed for a backyard flock. If you are raising them strictly to sell the eggs… then they are one of the best, usually laying over 300 large brown eggs per year per hen.

Fun fact: About 90% of the time, you can predict the color of the eggs a chicken will lay by the color of the earlobes. Chickens have a little tuft of feathers right over their ear sockets, and if white like the Leghorns, they will lay white eggs, and if brown or red the eggs will be brown.

Fancy Breeds:

These are usually not the best egg layers or meat birds, but are super fun and have great personalities.

Silkie: Silkies are known for their silky feathers that look like feather boas. The earliest recorded history of Silkies occurs in Marco Polo's writings about his travels to the Orient, and both China and Japan claim them as their country of origin. Their black skin and feathers, that feel a lot like silky hair, make them one of the most unusual varieties of chickens. Silkies come both bearded and non-bearded, and are excellent setters on all types of eggs. They are striking in appearance with their white plumage and mulberry colored comb, face, and wattles. The ear lobes are a light blue turquoise and the skin is dark bluish/black. In East Asia, they are considered a real meat delicacy.

Cochin: Cochins are known the world over for being big friendly balls of fluff and feathers. They don't lay well but are very popular because of their sweet personality and fantastic mothering qualities. Cochins became famous in the 1800s when this originally Chinese breed was given as a gift to Queen Victoria of England, who absolutely adored them.

Following the queen's lead, Cochins became a fad among poultry lovers in the English-speaking world, launching the breeding of fancy poultry in the west, as we know it today.

Cochins are one of the largest breeds, with cocks weighing up to 5 kg (11 lb.), and its soft and fluffy plumage, similar to the Japanese Silkie, exaggerates this bird's already large size.

Bantam: On the other side of the size spectrum from Cochins, Bantams are miniature chickens of several different breeds. You can have bantam cochins, bantam silkies, etc. Bantams are typically pretty aggressive.

Polish: The Polish or Poland is a European breed of chicken. The oldest documentation of these birds come from The Netherlands, but their exact origins are unknown. There are bearded, non-bearded and frizzle varieties. They are known for having a "furry head" due to not only having a v-shaped comb, but also a huge bouffant crest of feathers. This crest limits their vision, and as a result, though they are normally tame, they may be easily frightened and behave a bit wacky. When in a flock with more aggressive breeds, Polish will tend to be on the low end of the pecking order.

Polish chickens are bred today primarily as show birds, but were originally productive egg layers. Today, though, the breed produce inconsistent egg-layers, with some birds laying well, and some very poorly. In short, Polish are sweet, beautiful exhibition birds and can be good layers in the backyard flock, but they're not reliable producers.

Standard Care for Chickens:

There are a bunch of vaccinations, which are not usually state mandated, so some people don't do them. Good hatcheries will do them before they transport them, so you won't have to worry about the, but you will pay extra.

Flies, mites, and lice can be common in chickens, causing anemia or dermatitis.

Diet is very important to chickens, both to maintain health and to facilitate egg production. Because chickens have no teeth (hence the expression rare as hen's teeth) they don't actually chew their feed, so you need to ensure a source of grit (such as small pebbles, for example) either in the actual feed or the local environment, which can enter the gizzard. This is a muscular organ in the digestive tract, which harbors the grit, and via its mechanical action the grit in the gizzard "chews" the feed for the chicken, by grinding it up.

Adding calcium to the diet through oyster shell is also very important, as this will help strengthen and support the eggshell before the laying process. Oyster shell can be added to the feed each week, if needed. To save money, you can bake your used eggshells in the oven to dry them out, then crush them and add them to their feed, since the shells are full of calcium.

As you've read, animals to your farm can bring not only a lot of enjoyment, but can also be great food, fabric, service, or labor sources for your family, or even your market. Whichever animals you choose, if any, you should ensure that the costs of feeding, housing and maintaining them make economic sense when balanced against their return on investment, or understand that if not, you are intentionally choosing very expensive pets.

8. YOUR FARM AS YOUR BUSINESS

In this last section, we want to lead you through a process for deciding what you might want to do, vs. what worked for us, asking you to consider the following questions and suggestions, matched against your current skills, budget, and dreams.

You may want your farm to run as a big, profit generating concern. Or, you may want to have a fully sustainable, but small-scale operation that simply provides for your family's needs. You may want to have some interaction with a paying public, or minimize this as much as possible. You may not care if your farm does any of those things.

But in any case, you will need to generate some cash to pay for the things your farm can't provide, and which are needed to make it thrive, and/or to fulfill the revenue thresholds necessary to maintain a favorable tax status.

The following list is just a partial compilation of ideas and questions you could consider when deciding upon income sources for your farm, and remember, Google is your friend when you are trying to come up with ideas.

Income Sources:

If you are a teacher, have teaching experience, or just think you might like to teach, there is a huge need and yearning for any education about farming. We have been simply amazed at the number of people who want to learn, and realized, almost by accident, there was a business opportunity in this niche, which also is very different from what other farms in the area are offering.

Repurposing and Recycling: Olin is a master at repurposing and recycling and since he is a contractor, it's easy for him to come up with materials. He made our porch swing out of an antique door and left over building materials. It's easy to build, and we could charge $150-$200 just for the swing. If you included the frame to hang it on, you could sell that for $350 - $500 depending on the finishes. The antique door was salvaged from a house flip and the other materials cost was about $10, so the main cost is Olin's time. If you are not a contractor, you can still go to construction sites. If you see a construction site where they've discard materials, nine times out of ten they will let you take their scraps (but make sure you ask first). Lots of places have dumpsters sitting on the road.

Another repurposing example is using old windows, which Olin salvages from house flips, for art. Leigh is a painter and will paint roosters and farm scenes on the windows to sell at the farm. These windows range in price $100 - $150 each and provide Leigh a reason to continue her artwork, and customers with a unique painting from a local artist.

U-Pick Garden (or Pick Your Own): which we do. We cultivated close to 3 acres before we winnowed it down to around 2 acres. We only have a summer garden, but could easily have Spring and Fall Gardens too for more income. Our draw is the U-Pick Garden as a "drive to" destination. Then we get people to sign up to the newsletter (this becomes our "tribe")

Garden rentals: again, which we do. It's probably one of the most rewarding experiences, because you are helping families learn how to grow their own healthy food. It's empowering to be able to do that... kind of like giving a person a fish or teaching them to fish...they will never be hungry.

Sustainable Living Classes: which we also do. Remember when schools still had Home Economics Classes? All of those classes are now non-existent and families are hungry to learn the lost arts...canning, sourdough bread making, iron skillet cooking, bees and honey production and much more.

Petting Zoo: $20 per person. Sounds high, but when you walk into one, it's usually worth it. Need to decide if you want to be THAT open to the public.

Event Venue: Families and companies rent farms for all kinds of events now... Family Reunions, Birthday and Anniversary Parties, Weddings, fundraisers, corporate events and more. Unfortunately, our farm cannot be considered for weddings because of local code restrictions. Williamson County requires 20 acres to be able to host as a wedding venue, and we only have 15 acres.

Flower and Herb Farm: We grow flowers mainly to attract beneficial insects, but we end up selling quite a few for bouquets and arrangements. You could go as big as you want, selling for weddings and events. We also have Maximilian sunflowers that bloom in October and they are perfect for a wedding. Our summer flowers are cosmos, marigolds, buckwheat, zinnias and sunflowers. My favorite sales item is a flower and herb bouquet for $5 and the ladies love to pick them and do their own arrangement. We grow the big sunflowers all around the garden and we'll go pick those, and sell for $1 apiece. We sell the mammoth sunflowers for about $5 a head and customers can dry them for the sunflower seeds they yield.

Micro-Greens Farm: You can have a very small farm operation growing micro-greens for local restaurants. Most of the "up and coming" restaurants have sustainable chefs who want to BUY LOCAL. This is a growing business and can be done on a very small footprint.

Artist Farm: You could have a farm that entertains kids with fun programs and art themes. A great example is the Art Barn in Georgia, which you can find at the following URL: http://www.theartbarn.com/. Here is a description of the Art Barn on the website: "Atlanta's Best PRIVATE Barnyard & Farm Celebrations. Offering: Private Parties and Birthdays along with Group Events, Farm to Table Field Trips, Summer Camps, Afterschool Classes, Play dates, Educational Workshops & Seasonal Farm Fresh Goods and loads of Snuggling an amazing cast of critters. New Therapeutic Social Skills Groups and Orton Gillingham tutoring just added." Farmer Sue has cornered the market on kids' services revolving around an agriculture theme. We heard her speak at an Agritourism conference we attended and were very impressed.

Health/Fitness Farm: Imagine a picturesque farm with healthy food growing in raised beds, a 2 mile running track in a natural setting, outdoor and indoor workout equipment, personal trainers and yoga instructors leading individualized sessions, a refurbished barn/B&B, natural springs with a creek winding throughout the property.... wow, the possibilities!

Fish Farm: If your land has a large pond or lake, you could open a fish farm and allow people to come and enjoy an afternoon of fishing, while you collect income. Here is a website of one near us in Eagleville, TN: http://www.bluewatercatfishing.com/.

Survival Training/Shooting Range Farm: If your land is off the beaten path, away from neighborhoods, and zoned correctly you can provide services for local groups (Boy & Girl Scouts, personal trainers, corporate events and more). But remember, to continue a green belt status, you will need to make $1,500 per year in sales on hay, trees, fruit, vegetables or animals.

Pet Kennel/Pet Training Farm: Any size farm can have a kennel as the reason for the farm or a side operation for additional income. Borderland Farms has a large training facility for agility and diabetic alert dogs. The owner also rents some of her land to a local farmer who uses it for growing soybeans and other crops. We also have a state of the art Pet Kennel that houses and trains dogs and cats in Williamson County. You can research the spa-like atmosphere for your pet at the Farm at Natchez Trace:

http://thefarmatnatcheztrace.com/

Music Venue Farm: Have you heard of Woodstock, or more recently, Bonnaroo? Once a year the "Bonnaroo" farm is turned into a "destination" music venue and thousands of music lovers come from all over the United States to camp outside of Manchester, TN. Check out the Bonnaroo website for more information: http://www.bonnaroo.com/

Primitive Camping: If your land is "in the boonies" you can set up campsites (with or without electricity) by simply using landscape material and tree mulch (which you can get for free). Scouts and tourists love to frequent different places for their outings. You can even set up simple outdoor showers with rainwater capture. You will have to check your county's local compliance and zoning for this business idea.

Agritourism: Mazes, puzzles, treasure hunts for the kids (labyrinths), ghost walks, pumpkin patches (Mitchell Farm), haunted woods, zombie paintball hayrides, and zip lines are just some Agritourism ideas, and the sky's the limit. Families are always looking for somewhere to take the kids for the weekend or during the Summer.

Farm tours: We do a sustainability tour, for $5 a person, but require 20 people (so we can make at least $100 a tour). The walking tour takes an hour and we walk about 7 of the 15 acres on our farm. We cover composting, attracting beneficial insects, chickens, goats, rainwater capture, wetlands, blue line creek, and more. At first, we did not require 20 people, but we had to have set a limit, because otherwise you will work yourself to death. We target cub scouts, girl scouts, home school groups (that's Leigh's main one) and church groups. We don't market to public schools because we would have to hire employees to help with much larger groups.

Each child receives a sustainable farm tour map and booklet designed by a former farm intern and TSU graduate student, Sarah Hovis. Sarah included games about beneficial insects, farm animals, wetlands and much more. It's not only fun but also very educational.

Raised Bed Gardens: Olin has actually built 4'x4' or 4'x8' raised bed gardens for people and delivers them for a fee. This is not a huge moneymaker, but if you add some additional services, like assisting them in designing and planting the garden, it could be worthy.

Bed and Breakfast: This can be a great revenue stream for a rural property. You have to consider how you will check out (vet) people who will be staying at your home, how they will pay you, and what requirements you will need as far as deposits, cancellation policy, etc. Depending on local codes, you may have to register and license your B&B. Lots to consider.

Speaking engagements (off-site): Joel Salatin with Polyface farms in Virginia charges $2000 plus expenses to give any type of speaking engagements he goes to. Speakers charge anywhere from $1,500 to $20K or more for people in the agriculture field. Check out this speaker's bureau website for more information: http://agriculturalspeakers.com/. What you can charge depends on how big your tribe is, how popular you are, etc.

The Salatins are a family who moved to Virginia in 1961 and now 55 years later the farm hosts 4 generations. Inspiring and expanding the notion of sustainable farming the world over to such an extent that they have become the subject of a film.

Farm Conferences: Each year (or multiple times) you can host a conference to share with others, your expertise. We host a Sustainable Living Farm Conference each year in the Spring before the U-Pick Garden begins, and share how to grow your own healthy food, live sustainably, and have multiple income streams while you are living your dream. How much you can charge per person or per couple is dependent on the knowledge/skills you are sharing as well as your popularity in the marketplace.

Educational Products: You can reach more people through the internet, if you have a product that educates others on your particular expertise. Some people offer a DVD, an e-book, or a downloadable learning program. Others offer free information in exchange for your e-mail address subscription. Regardless of the product you choose, this is a great income stream and method to build your "tribe".

Product sales: Hats, aprons with logos, cookbooks, notecards, and cute farm t-shirts are all fun things you can sell in your store or online. Leigh also sells jam, jelly and apple butter. (In the Fall, she makes about 200 jars of muscadine jelly at one time, freezes the leftover grapes and then continues to make smaller batches on an ongoing basis, as demand requires). She sells each half pint jar for $5 each. Sour dough bread ($5) and cinnamon rolls ($8) are more seasonal and made to order (except during the summer when she makes it readily available). Another product is gift baskets at Christmas with homemade jams and jellies and bread or cinnamon rolls, for corporate accounts. Orders can be worth $200 - $500 each (with multiple baskets per order). She recently made an order for a local Realtor for 20 caramel cakes to deliver around Groundhog Day as a "thank you" for his customers.

Green House Rental: If you have a greenhouse, or if you want to build a temporary greenhouse, you can rent space to organizations or individuals who want to grow their garden plants from seeds. For two years in a row, we rented part of our greenhouse to the Williamson County Master Gardener's Association, and grew plants for several people in the community.

Consulting: Many years of sustainable living on the farm has afforded us the opportunity to help others create their own self-sufficient life. Olin has 30-plus years of experience in the construction and engineering field which helps him consult on any type of sustainable housing project. We have assisted numerous families and individuals on the best use of their land, where to launch their farm, and even income sources. We have provided resources for tapping into natural springs, fencing, soil testing, and septic. Sustainable Consulting includes an in-person walk through of the farm and a detailed report on recommendations and resources. If you have a similar skill set, consulting can provide a solid side income.

Educational Classes: Largely due to the lack of Home Economics classes in the school system, there is a huge gap in life skills such as preserving food and so much more. Some of the classes we offer are:

1) Probiotic-rich Kefir and Kombucha: We actually provide the kefir grains, and Kombucha Scobie to get people started on their own batch. The class demonstrates the different stages of fermentation as well as flavoring to taste.

2) Canning 101: Preserving food for winter months is part of the sustainable lifestyle. Leigh teaches, pressure and water bath canning, blanching for the freezer, jams/jellies, pickling, and dried food. This is the longest of all the classes and lasts 2 hours. Your audience (and possibly you!) will lose interest after 2 hours.

3) Healthy Juicing: Juicing has become a very important change in Healthy diets. Some people do it for the enzymes and vitamins and others do it to help control symptoms of autoimmune diseases.

4) Protecting and Preserving our Local Pollinators: The global bee population is diminishing, and every community has a responsibility to protect and preserve them. This class teaches important facts about our pollinators and the details of having your own hive (either now or in the future).

5) Quick and Easy Healing Meals: With families "on the go," and less time to eat together, these meals are easy and fast ways to provide real nutrition during the week. Imagine your family getting really tasty vegetarian meals instead of the predictable pizza or Happy Meal.

6) Gardening 101: Basics of gardening, soil testing, growing from seed, transplanting, rainwater capture, composting.

7) Cooking Classes: We hold several of these each year varying from ethnic food to vegetarian and everything in between. We usually host a local chef.

8) Painting or Art Classes: We host local art teachers or Leigh will teach. Mediums include canvas or recycled windows with acrylic paint.

9) Sustainable Wreath Making: Every December we have a wreath making class that our Aunt Eloise Corley leads. She does a terrific job in showing people how to make handmade wreaths out of cedar branches, pine-cones and other sustainable components. This is one of our most popular classes!

10) Sustainable Kids Crafts: Kids love to create and who would have thought that we would find so many different ways to use a piece of dried okra? We've made Okra Angels, Okra Butterflies and Okra Grasshoppers to name a few. We have also made crafts with birdhouse gourds…there is no limit to what you can create.

Leigh often hosts speakers, and will split everything down the middle, which includes their supplies. So for instance, if the class is $35 per person and the speaker/teacher bought $50 of supplies, then Leigh takes those expenses out of the total revenue, and then divides it down the middle. Leigh's venue fee is half of it, and the speaker fee is half plus the cost of supplies.

In general, Leigh tries to generate at least $150 in income per class, so she will market the classes though Social Media and a community-advertising site called Hob Nob Franklin, to ensure an appropriate amount of participation. If Leigh is teaching the class @ $35 per person, then her minimum is 5 people. If she hosts a speaker, then she would need at least 10 people to make the same amount. We would advise that you decide how much income you want to receive to make it worth your while. You just don't make enough money if you do classes for only a few people. Your time has value and you can always reschedule the class for another date, if you don't get enough response.

As mentioned earlier, Leigh is a painter, so the art classes suits her need for creativity in her work. You have to remember that each income stream still needs to focus on your mission; don't get too crazy. For her everything revolves around the model of sustainability, so sunflowers (adults) and ladybugs (kids) are some of the themes she has chosen for painting classes.

The main goal of educational or art classes is to enrich the lives of the people in the community, as well as focus on the mission of our farm.

Whatever you decide to do, we'd highly encourage you to find passionate people who want to help you. They are out there and you both will be richer for it.

If you are dependent on the income, then of course you need to find the income streams that will work for you. But you should also have a longer-term strategy where you can begin to focus not only on maximizing income but also feeding your heart, so that you are doing things that fuel your passion.

As we've said, our passion has become teaching some of the things that we have learned by living a sustainable life. And the great advantage of that is the continual learning each and every day. We don't just share our knowledge, we learn from others constantly as they share their ideas and successes.

Think About Outsourcing:

If there is a service, product, or experience something you can't or don't want to provide yourself, but you do want to have it on your farm, you can just outsource it. The well-known recording artist: Kix Brooks, is part owner of Arrington Vineyards, in Franklin, TN. Kix knows music, but when he started didn't know a whole lot about producing wine. By providing a live music venue, Arrington supports local music artists, and by outsourcing the wine production and marketing, is making a lot of money doing so.

Other forms of outsourcing could be 1) renting your land to other farmers to raise crops, 2) renting land/stalls for a horse boarding business, and 3) renting space for survival training, a gun range or maybe a fitness endurance venue (check out http://soaradventure.com).

There's not a whole lot of money in "farming" as in, producing food. But certain cash crops (hops, hemp) can make you a lot of money. You should still farm for your own needs, as that is more sustainable, but there a lot of other ways to make money from your farm.

General Tips for staying sane:

We'd advise not trying to do too much at once. Also, give yourself room to make mistakes (maybe not destroying 2/3 of the tomato crop by over-fertilizing, but you know, mistakes.) When starting out, take things a little at a time; figure out your interests, what you like to do, what will give a reasonable return on the output of your effort and time (as in, not hosting a tour for five people, because that is just as much work as hosting one for 20 people).

At least locally, be the best at (or as good as everyone else) at the service or product you are offering. Try not to overcommit yourself, or spread yourself too thin. We slowed down after that first year, because we were killing ourselves, and that's when we intentionally said to each other: "hey, we don't want this to become another corporate job!" It's quite possible we were too used to that pace, and needed to unlearn some of those behaviors, and you may have some "unlearning" to do as well.

Unlearning some of the behaviors that you bring to the farming lifestyle may include understanding that there are different rhythms to things than the one demanded by a corporate machine. Things really do happen in their season, not everything has to happen with an outsized sense of urgency. You will discover that there really are only so many hours in the day, and not everything can be done today. Your priorities will shift so that the some important things can wait until the most important and urgent things have been taken care of. You will come to know that not everything is equally urgent and important, which the corporate mindset can trick you into believing.

We were open every day, and aggressively marketing our farm, and we have to admit that this activity did generate us a list of over 1,000 people that we could add to our email list. And it is true of every business that "your money is in your list."

But this pace meant that our garden couldn't yield enough produce to handle the demand we would get. By the weekend, we'd be out of stuff that we could sell, which is not a position you want to find yourselves. Limiting our "open" times allowed us to have enough output to meet our customer's demands, and feel a lot less stressed, while making the same amount of money.

How much money do you want and need to earn?

Leigh made over 6 figures in the corporate world. So the big question was whether we could do without her income. First we became debt free. Then we could envision what else we could do by budgeting, living more simply, buying fewer clothes, etc.

Olin: "The first thing we did was to pay for all the kids college. As any parent knows, there are lots of sacrifices behind the scenes that your children do not know you do." Previously Olin was one of those who lived on the credit card edge, keeping up with the Joneses, but not anymore.

Business Funnel:

Every business needs multiple sources of income. For instance, a well-known local company, the Lee Company, now does multiple services. They started out doing HVAC, then progressed to plumbing, and now do remodeling and electrical work. On a small farm, especially, you should have diverse sources of income.

However, you also have to be careful not to get away from your core competencies, and your ability to manage several different types of services. So if you don't like it, and aren't interested in it, it is unlikely you will manifest the necessary follow through to implement it properly. But if you only have one income funnel, then when demand for that service wanes, you are stuck. Having more than one funnel around your core competence and mission is important. Keep in mind too, how much time you are spending on each source of income. It's fun to make and sell jams and jellies, but classes and events are much better income streams, in terms of Internal ROI.

When you start your business, we would advise to pick a niche, no more than 2-3, built around your core competency, passion, and mission, so that you do not diminish focus.

Leigh was three years into the farm before she started making sourdough bread. She got her Aunt Susan Willis' 1990 recipe/sourdough starter, and began making bread and teaching classes. Then she said, "man, if I can sell this bread, that'd be awesome." So she does. It's quite a bit of work, but she loves it, and you make $5 for a pan of rolls, and $5 for a loaf of bread.

Leigh and two volunteers, Sarah Cho and Kendall Pinkston, made over $1,100 making bread one summer at the U-Pick Garden. It was a ton of work, and the internal rate of return (revenue received for time, effort and expense put in) was probably not enough, but they loved doing it. She used the money to take Sarah and Kendall (surrogate daughters) on a trip to Universal Studios in Florida, as a thank you for all their help.

She paints, (and sells paintings,) but makes more money teaching painting classes out at the farm.

We know this business model can yield $25-30K a year, but Leigh, who is retired, doesn't work even close to a full time schedule, because she wants to devote a lot of her time to volunteer work.

But remember, our farm goal is not all about the money, and Olin has a full-time job outside of the farm. Olin currently owns a company with three other partners and they are working for their eventual retirement. His company is part of our retirement portfolio, so the urgency to make money on the farming operation is not as great as if it was the only source of revenue.

Olin makes the monthly money to take care of living, expenses, so that Leigh's farm income can be supplemental for luxuries (such as vacations, e.g.).

So Leigh can indulge her passion with her mission. A lot of it is lifestyle and flexibility. This past year she had a very good friend who was terminally ill, and she spent a lot of quality time with her over the last 4-5 months of her life. In the corporate world she would not have had the opportunity to be there for her friend.

When Olin leaves his current full time day job and can join in the revenue side of the farm, his skills with recycling and repurposing (e.g. selling swings from discarded building materials) will really increase the farm income. He is very talented at woodworking and repurposing is a passion for him, so this will fit not only what he loves to do, but will also offer up another educational area for him to teach, if he wants to.

We understand that your economic reality may be different, and may require that the bulk of your income come from your farm. But someone who really wanted to build a healthy income stream from a farm-related niche could easily make $50 – 100K or more... depending on the time and effort they wanted to invest. A large Agritourism farm, for instance, can make $100K+ profit per year.

When you start a new business venture, and a farm is no different, you should consider it will take a solid two years before you see a real profit, so you need working capital to live on and cover expenses for that time. Therefore you either need a partner who has a full-time income, a residual income from another source, or savings that will carry you through that two-year period (or some combination of the above).

Exit Strategies:

When you have a business, at some point you are going to need to think about your exit strategy. When you first start out, this probably won't be high on your to-do list, which is understandable.

But once you are up and running, your revenue streams may or may not contribute a whole lot to the value of your business, because when someone buys your business they are basically paying for the revenue streams (and book value of assets) that they can capture without YOU being there. So every revenue stream that is dependent on you being there is not contributing to the overall value of the business from a buyer's perspective. Suppose you have some special, unique skill that generates revenue for the business. Because this is not reproducible income without you there, it is irrelevant to them when they buy you out, because they can't duplicate it with you gone.

So, you can try to lay out a how-to manual, if it is a teachable thing, but if it's not, or if they know they aren't going to do it because it doesn't fit THEIR passion, then it's discounted when they go to buy you out.

When we said earlier, the money is in the list, what that really means is the value of your business is in your customer base, and how many of those customers can be retained by the one-day buyer of your business. Yes, you are essentially selling your "list" of customers.

Your leadership strategy is to plan for the day you are not there. So Leigh and Olin's goal is not to leave the farm business to their kids, because they (the kids) do not want to run a teaching farm.

You could decide just to close the business and sell the land, or you can sell as a viable business, so you will need to know what it is you are selling. A great way to determine the 'book value' of your business is to seek help from a business broker, who can help you determine the actual amount someone would be willing to pay for your "list" and assets.

At least for now, though, our mission centers around teaching people how to grow their own healthy food, it's not about making money. For instance, we have sold nearly double the berries last year than we did the year before, just because so many people seem to want a place to come and pick berries.

But we are not going to turn ourselves into a big, specialized, berry-producing combine. That doesn't fit the mission, nor in fact is it congruent with the "sustainable farming" concept. The purpose of the U-Pick Garden is to teach families where their food comes from, and to take them out of the rat race for short time. With so many families having two working parents, kids in sports, and a week full of non-stop activities, it's nice having a place to relax, sit and rock on the porch, visit the chickens and goats, and have some down time.

An interesting story we like to tell is that our volunteer, Sarah Cho, found Stoney Creek BECAUSE we grew a variety of vegetables and fruit in the U-Pick Garden. She went online to find u-pick farms, one focused just on strawberries, another was a pumpkin patch, and a couple of blueberry farms, but she was not interested in any of those. She wanted to find out more about our "vegetable garden" and joined as an intern. Sarah still feels like she is learning, because she will start her third year assisting us at the farm. She and her husband, Kung He, are like family to us.

Marketing Your Farm:

Having a website is a given. You can do these very inexpensively now, especially using Wordpress. Be careful whom you use to create your website (if you don't do it yourself), as you can needlessly spend a lot of money.

It's very important to have a contact form on your website, to gather an email list. You also need a blog, a Facebook page, Twitter, Pinterest, Instagram and a presence on LinkedIn. Facebook "LIVE" is a feature for the live broadcast of user videos from the Facebook Mobile App. If you are comfortable talking to people 'on the fly', there is good reason to use this app. Live video is heavily weighted on the Google Search Engine and increases the chance of being seen by more people. Not everyone has a YouTube channel, but we feel this is a great way to communicate and educate your audience. Our YouTube channel is called 'Stoney Creek Farm' and can be searched at www.youtube.com. All of these methods will help you communicate with your growing 'tribe' of followers.

Your website should also be mobile friendly, as Google reports that 70% of its searches are now done via a mobile device. The latest version of Wordpress automatically makes your site-mobile-friendly. If you already have a website, you can test it for mobile friendliness at this free Google URL:

https://www.google.com/webmasters/tools/mobile-friendly/

Write a Book:

When you share what you do in public, whether it's at a seminar or even in casual conversation, people will nod and say, oh that was interesting, but as soon as you write it down and put it into paper, digital or audio form, your credibility goes through the roof because now you have written a book.

Our author friend Paul Deepan likes to say: "It's no mystery why the words "author" and "authority" have the same root. If you "author" a book, you will be considered an "authority" on that subject, no matter what it is." As farming educators, part of the reason for authoring this book is that our credibility on the subject will be enhanced, and people will be more willing to sign up for our seminars because we have written a book.

There are many ways to promote yourself as an author. As a start, you can go to the local library (and lots of libraries promote local authors) and say: I've got a book! Then you give a little presentation at the library or local bookstore, or wherever.

People will think you know what you are talking about far more than they did before. If you can breathe your personal journey into where and how you got to where you are, why you're doing what you are doing, this will greatly help to share your passion to the world, so it becomes more interesting to read, and more widely shared and recommended. Despite all the technological ways of marketing yourself, writing a book is still really, really powerful. And even in our digital age, it's still the number one thing that will position you the fastest as an expert in your field.

As an example, Dave Ramsey, in *Financial Peace*, talks about his early financial struggles and how that evolved into his passion to help himself and others how to become debt free and live in Peace from a financial perspective. His techniques are interesting, but his application of them to his own life when he was in financial difficulties is what make them compelling.

You will not likely make a lot of money on your book sales (which is why we didn't include this section under "Revenue Streams." Your book is rather used as a marketing tool to drive your credibility in your business, which helps you command more money for speaking fees, to promote your niche, and build your audience.

Archive your list of events, your blog posts, etc. This can all be fodder for longer, specialized articles, and/or eventually developed into your book. The average book should be a minimum 20,000 words, better at over 40,000 words, max should be no longer than 60,000, depending on your audience and interest in your topic.

If you do want commercial sales of your book, you can research what topics are "hot" in Amazon by using Google Ad words, and testing frequency of those ad words in title searches in Amazon Kindle. Any titles with those keywords that rank above # 100,000 (either in category or across Amazon Kindle) could be good candidates for a book topic. Paul Deepan has access to software which actually tracks sales rankings and unit sales of Kindle e-books by category; feel free to connect with him if you'd like more information about this topic (www.mycontentmatters.net).

If you want your book to be a giveaway as part of building your authority platform, then this kind of pre-publication market research is not as essential. Using this strategy, your book sales will not typically become a significant revenue stream, but you will definitely build credibility in your niche if you have published a book-length manuscript.

If you aren't a writer, there are many ways to inexpensively outsource blog, articles, and even book writing, editing, and publishing services that we would be happy to share if you got in touch.

Make sure to collect post-event commentary on event/class, with comments from participants. This is a great way to gather contact information, and follow up to ensure interest in future classes.

Affiliate Marketing:

Consider becoming an affiliate marketer on your website for products that align with your vision and mission. These can be anything from informational products like books and DVD's etc., to favorite supplies, tools, etc. that you'd endorse to a friend. It's possible to earn anywhere from 10-50% commission from the authors/suppliers of these items via their sales on your website, because you are generating new customers for them to whom they would not otherwise be visible or accessible.

The plug-ins necessary to track that visitors to your site are buying their products are easy to install, especially if you are using a Wordpress site, and if you are organically driving enough traffic to your site via your blogs, Facebook posts, and email engagement programs, this can become a fairly lucrative passive income stream.

Sometimes individual people/companies may not affiliate with you unless you can demonstrate a certain amount of traffic to your website, but this is not as much of an obstacle as it used to be, and certainly if you set up as an Amazon affiliate, they won't worry about this, and will in fact give you tips and strategies to help you generate traffic. Almost anything you can think of selling as an affiliate on your farm website is probably available on Amazon anyway, so this could be an excellent place to start with such a program.

If you are an affiliate (for example with Amazon) and someone buys a product that they see on your site that is an Amazon product offering, Amazon will accept payment and do the order fulfillment for you, so you don't have to keep physical inventory of the things you are selling as an affiliate in your garage, or barn, or anything like that. If the customer buys something you are offering yourself, then you would of course have to have the inventory on hand to fulfill the order, and give them a way to pay you online.

Affiliate marketing can be a lucrative additional income to your farm business, or even for other interests you may have outside of your farm passion. Just be aware that there is a lot of competition out there, and you almost certainly won't see a lot of money from this activity, certainly not in the beginning, and it's definitely not the path to quick riches. So we'd advise you focus on your main passion within the farming activity itself, and against making this the main income stream for your farm business. But it can develop over a period of several years into something that is quite profitable, and not very time-consuming to maintain.

Taking Online Payments:

We are not endorsing PayPal, but this is the payment system we use, and they charge a fee per transaction. It is a very convenient way of accepting payments online. Even if the customer does not have a PayPal account, they can still pay with a credit card via PayPal. You need to track your transaction fees, as these are tax-deductible expenses of doing business, but just be aware that PayPal doesn't always make it easy to find how much you are paying them per transaction. There are a number of credit card processing firms, some of which specialize in online marketing, so it would be wise to look at several before deciding which one is right for your business model.

Building Your List:

You should aim to eventually have at least 3-5000 people on your mailing list. Facebook limits the number of people an individual can have as "friends" to 5000 people. So you should register your farm as a BUSINESS Facebook site to allow yourself more than 5000 followers. You can't change your designation, and you can't take the people you already have over to a new site, you will have to ask them to like you on your new page all over again, so make sure you avoid this mistake (which we made) when you are starting out.

What you need for your email list: Subscribe to newsletter or blog (have this on front page). You will want to list a couple of benefits to this for joining like "Be the first to get news of upcoming events, early bird discounts, etc.)" Only ask for a first name and email address (more info required the less likely they are to fill out). You will need their first name to personalize future e-mail to them. The first name is important because you can get some pretty weird email addresses, for example like rocketship49@.mail.net, and you don't want to send out an email saying "Dear Rocketship49."

Networking groups:

Networking is important for all businesses. We joined BNI (Business Networking International, which claims it is the largest business networking organization in the world). This costs roughly $1,000 for the first year, inclusive of organization registration, and quarterly chapter dues.

BNI members can join by invitation only (have to be sponsored) and you will be the only person in your industry in that Chapter. Visit more than one group to ensure you are a fit.

At the time, Leigh needed to double her gross income, so the farm was not considered as a 'hobby'. If you sell locally, you'd want to join a group like that, as it is an effective and high quality way to connect with people in your area. Networking relationships can take a while to build, so your networking group may not generate a ton of revenue for you right away, but over time it can be a very good source of word-of-mouth referral business, from people who have come to know you.

Your local Chamber of Commerce Organization may also be a good for fit for your business networking opportunities.

Events:

Gatherings like our annual Farm Conference must be marketed at least 6 months to a year to draw enough participation. Other events, like classes, may only need one month to 6 weeks of marketing. We have tried to plan our classes for the whole year (or even for 3 months at a time), but for whatever reason, we are more successful marketing closer to the event date. We have also found that class dates and speaker's schedules invariably change, and we ended up rescheduling about half the classes when we tried to plan ahead.

Farm Associations are a wonderful way to keep abreast of industry trends and network with other farms. We have attended the Tennessee Agritourism Conference for years and it really opened our eyes to what revenue streams were possible. It would also be fun and educational to attend those types of conferences in nearby states.

Online Advertising:

We use a local community ad site, called Hob Nob Franklin. Users are allowed to blog on the site once each day, and over 50,000 people in the Franklin area see our posts. They charge a very reasonable monthly advertising fee and you control all the posts. All of my classes are listed on the site, as well as blog posts that I also repeat on my website. Hob Nob also automatically links posts to Social Media, like Twitter and Facebook, so you don't have to post each individually. Hob Nob has other community sites throughout the United States, just check out www.hobnoblocal.com.

Leigh does not do LinkedIn ads, because she believes that they "haven't gotten it yet:" the one ad she posted, did not do well and the ads are expensive.

Leigh DOES do Facebook Ads (not a whole lot, about $400 last year, mostly advertising her conference). Go to Ads Manager, and you can pick your budget. You will want less than 17c. You can Google how to post an ad on Facebook, so we will not go into great detail here, but you want < 17c.

One ad Leigh recently posted reached 1,000 people, with 71 responses, mostly likes. But she only spent $5. If you mimic this, you will then now who these folks are, so you can connect with them subsequently. When you do this follow up, basically just say thanks for liking the post, and if you want, you can also ask them to friend you/follow your page on FB. That way, they will get notifications about other posts you make on FB. If you have a business page, a like will automatically become a follower, but still follow up and say thanks. If you still have a personal page, you will need to proactively do the follow-up.

As in email marketing, don't go all hard sell with social media. The point is to inform, and possibly entertain, NOT sell. If they find the info useful, they will come to you, refer to you, etc. The general rule of thumb is 80% sharing and 20% selling.

You can target ads to a specific geographic radius and different interests such as 'homesteading' and 'mother earth news'.

Twitter (140 character messages) and Instagram (pictures) can also be very useful social media platforms.

Using your local newspaper can be a very effective way to get publicity, often for free, if you for instance offer to do an article for them that you can show has relevance to their readership.

We've had three newspapers come out and do articles on the farm, and the same thing happened with a local TV channel looking for an interesting human interest story. You will be able to these video segments and post them on your website. We were fortunate to have our local PBS station cover a segment on our farm for Volunteer Gardener and that show is listed on our website. Local station (WZTV) Fox 17 covered us on a segment in one of their newscasts and Christian Broadcast Network included us in a segment with Dan Miller (48days.com). We have been blessed.

We also won the 2014 innovative marketing award for small farmers in Tennessee, awarded by the TSU Cooperative Extension. Getting involved with your local Agriculture Extension office will help in getting your farm recognized in the community and state.

We would definitely suggest reading Guerilla Marketing by Jay Conrad Levinson, and check out which marketing ideas are right for your business. You can get a lot of ideas on how to market your farm for free.

Marketing to Health and Fitness networks may benefit your reach in the community (you are promoting a healthier lifestyle by having a farm). Visit every chiropractor, because they can refer people to you very easily. Also Nutritionists, vitamin shops, personal trainers, yoga instructors and massage therapists are often good contacts. You can offer a referral fee if one of their referrals comes to an event, etc.

Leigh does NOT do Groupon, and here is why: You put ad on Groupon, usually a 50% discount. Groupon gets 50% of what's left, so you get 25% of what you'd get otherwise, and this makes no financial sense to Leigh. Groupon erodes profitability, but does not build a loyal customer base (in other words, the kind of people you attract through Groupon will be the kind of customers who will only come once when you offer a Groupon, not because they intrinsically value you, your farm, or your services).

You have to "market" for people to help you work on the farm too. We use volunteers, as mentioned previously. Typically, intern volunteers will only be there for a single season, so you do have to recruit more every year. But two of our interns (Sarah and Kendall) have hung around because there is so much they want to learn. Sarah's husband has a good job, and Kendall has a full time job which permits them the freedom to volunteer at the farm. They learn how to make sourdough, can veggies, make jams, grow the food, plus they receive a lot of the produce and product generated by farm operations for free, which lowers their own weekly food budgets. They are also able to go to any of the classes they choose for free (unless there is a guest speaker, then they pay only the speaker fee).

Your marketing is extremely critical. It's critical for every business, and very few small business owners, in particular, do enough of it. Some research suggests that if you are a small business, 60-70% of your time should be spent marketing, which is the reverse of what most people do, because they feel they don't have the time to do that much because they are so busy doing the operations part of their business.

Most people get caught up in the operational piece, because that is what they are good at, and often why they started their business in the first place. Then the marketing of the business tends to fall by the wayside, which ultimately becomes a problem, because all of a sudden when there is a lull in customer growth (not if, when, it nearly always happens), decline in demand, etc., you can find yourself really struggling for revenue.

Make time to market your business. Even if it feels you don't have time to do it, you aren't good at it, whatever, make the time to do it, or at least outsource this function, to get help with it.

Ideally you should be posting a blog to your site as frequently as three times a week, and promoting the blog/article, etc. out to your tribe via email and your social media platforms. If you can't make three times a week, then either hire someone to do that for you, or at minimum post once a week, preferably on Monday. There is nothing that says you aren't engaged with your clients more than having a blog on your website and the last post being six months ago, or longer.

It will take at least six touches before someone will make a buying decision, and digital engagement is no different, so you have to be steadily engaged with your tribe so that they will be loyal and eventually "buy" from you. They will get upset with you if you are just trying to sell them all the time, which is why your blog content and emails, etc., should be non-promotional in nature, informative, and not trying to sell people. You must give away valuable relevant free content.

Just as it might take you several tries to discover what your actual passion is for your farm, and what activities provide the best return on your investment from a business standpoint, so too will your marketing efforts take a little time to refine. What we are trying to do here is give you some tools that we know have worked for us, so that hopefully some of this marketing effort is less hit and miss on the front end.

Growing your sales can happen without a lot of increase in expenses. For example, hosting a painting class for 20 people may cost you a little more in terms of supplies, than if you held a class for only 5 people, but your time investment is the same, and the total amount of money you make, as well as profits, are much higher.

So if I figure out that my time is worth, say $50 per hour, that means the time and expense I put in marketing and delivering a 3 hour class should net me about $150, minimum. Which means if I hold a class for $35 for a 3-hour session, I need at minimum 6-7 people there, to compensate me for my material costs, time spent marketing, and time spent giving the class.

The 3 c's: Competence, Capacity and Capital. Do I know how to do it? DO I have the time/space to do it? DO I have the financial, emotional, physical reserves to do it?

You can make a ton of money and hate it (like say you leave a high paying corporate job to start a farm). So if you don't like it you probably won't stick with it. If it's a passion, you don't feel like it's work at all!

9. LAST WORDS

What did we wish we knew before we started?

That's perhaps the most important question this book is trying to help you answer.

Fact: Farming is a lot of really hard, physically demanding work!

But, if you let yourself have enough fun with it, the rewards are amazing.

Just remember, that even with a resource like this book, it's inevitable (and important) that you will make mistakes, and have miscommunication… it's just part of the learning experience.

It might have been nice to know that what Olin meant when he asked Leigh to "Please fertilize the tomatoes, with a handful of fertilizer," was for her to use that handful for an entire row, and not every plant.

It might also have been nice to know that our mission was to grow healthy food, and to teach others how to do the same, earlier than we came to that discovery.

But I don't think either of us would trade any of the hard-earned lessons that we went through by facing all these situations, and coming through them together. We hold our sense of mission with conviction precisely because it had such a long and complex gestation. We became creative with how we used our farm because we did not want to be in competition with sister farms and our interests were very different from traditional farming.

We have grown into an unshakeable belief that the work we do here is really a ministry of faith, an acknowledgment of God beyond the limits of any one religion. Our beliefs have sustained us through the ups and downs of life and we recognize how hungry so many of our visitors are to get back to the land, even if they've never so much as held a shovel in their hands. It's very rewarding to see how satisfied they appear, if even for just the brief time they are with us, to have spent that time outdoors, in God's own cathedral, close to the living treasure that is his soil, basking in the abundance that His garden provides.

We are Dirt Rich indeed.

ABOUT THE AUTHORS

Leigh Funderburk was born in Humboldt, Tennessee, and has lived in the state for most of her life. She graduated from Middle Tennessee State University with a BS in psychology, and had an extensive 30-year corporate career, most recently with Xerox, before "going back to the farm." She retired from corporate life in 2013, to better devote her energy to sustainable farming.

Olin Funderburk was born in Biloxi, Mississippi, and, as a "preacher's kid," lived all over the Southeast. Olin has a BS in Construction, Engineering, and Technology from the University of Southern Mississippi, and currently owns a construction company with three other partners, where he still works.

Olin and Leigh have been teaching people how to live a more simple and sustainable life since they opened Stoney Creek Farm to the public in 2010. Their dream is to help everyone become "Dirt Rich," whether they live in the country or the city.

~

Paul Deepan was born in Port-of-Spain, Trinidad, and in addition to the United States, has lived in Trinidad, England and Canada. He received his undergraduate degree from the University of Toronto, and Master's degrees in Biology and Business from the Universities of Waterloo, and Western Ontario, respectively. Paul is the author of the award-winning fantasy novel, *The Fruit of the Dendragon Tree*, and has written and taught in a variety of niches, including fiction: (short stories, poems, and songs), and non-fiction: (monographs and case studies, etc. in marketing, finance, and health care). Paul ghost writes book-length projects for people who may be too busy or too overwhelmed to tackle this daunting task on their own. He deeply values his friendship with Leigh and Olin, and the labor of love that became *Dirt Rich*. He visits Stoney Creek Farm whenever possible, and believes that everybody should.